Most advertising in the world pertaining to health and nutrition is baseless in its claims which is why the FDA has begun a major crackdown on such advertising. Most if not all ads for drugs start off talking about how wonderful the drug is and what it can prevent and then a picture of a cute little puppy or kitten appears while they go through a lengthy list of side effects or should I say direct effects of that drug, ranging from stroke, heart failure to nothing short of blindness and paralysis. Well just sign me up for that drug.

By the time you finish this book and read it again for a second time you will have a pretty good understanding of what will or won't work for you specifically. You see, my philosophy has always been "we are all biochemically different" so what works for one person may not work for the other when it comes to food and supplements. For one person to come out and say we were all meant to be vegetarians or mixed carnivores is as ridiculous as me saying we should all be wearing a size 9 shoe. It just isn't so.

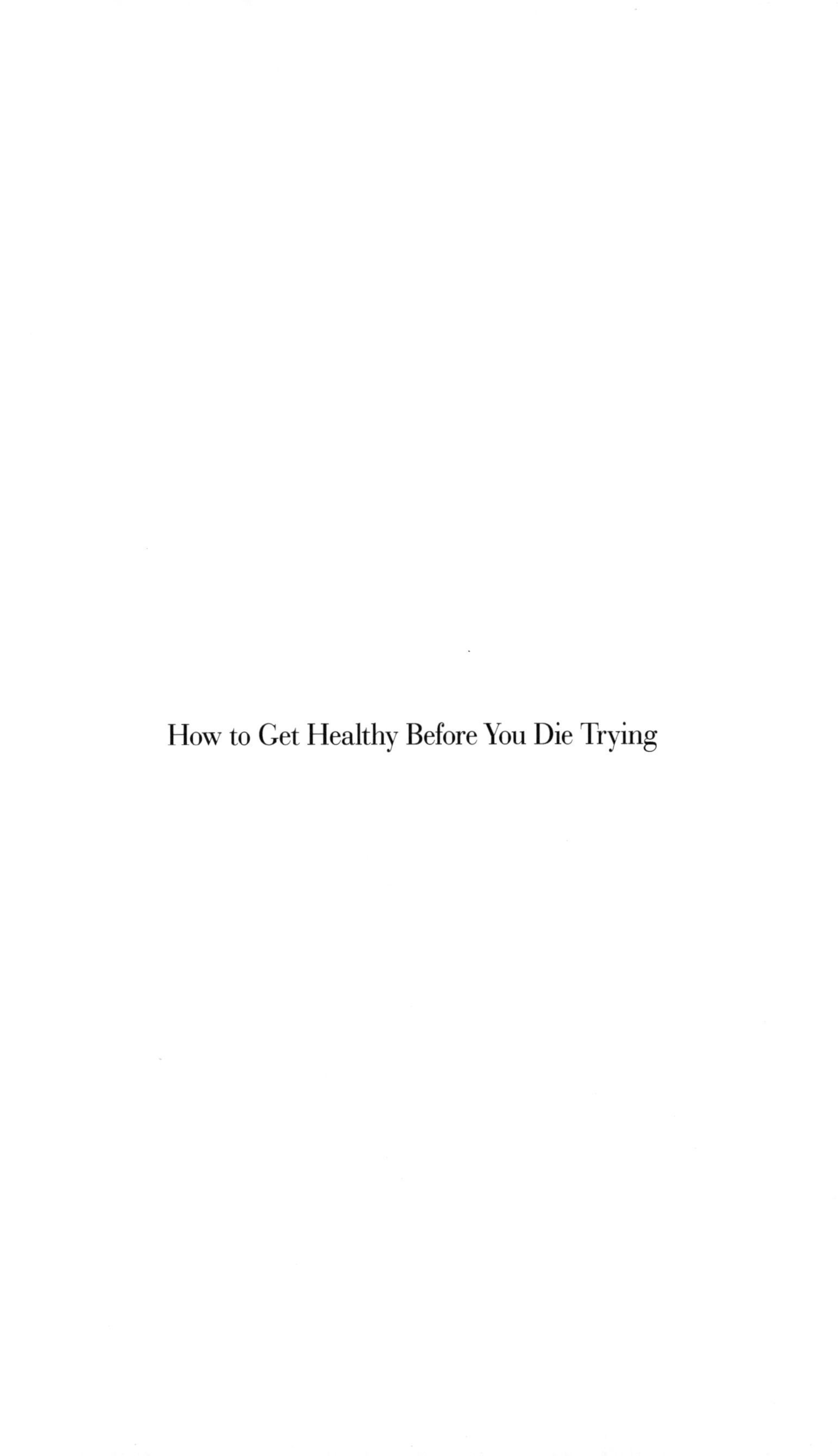

How to Get Healthy Before You Die Trying

Tell Me, Teach Me, Heal Me

How to Get Healthy Before You Die Trying

Douglas Caporrino

ISBN: 978-1-4834-9736-5 (sc)
ISBN: 978-1-4834-9735-8 (e)

Lulu Publishing Services rev. date: 04/23/2019

Contents

Dedication

For My Mom:

We have all heard the phrase "Knowledge is Power" but I would extend that phrase to "Action is Influence".

Had I known then what I know now I might have prevented many of my mom's many surgeries or painful years of suffering. She was a woman who endured countless surgeries, over 20. Four total hip replacements, several back surgeries, several abdominal surgeries due to complications from her hip surgeries, a shoulder surgery here and there and a few bouts with cancer.

Countless years of pain killers that created direct effects of stomach problems, sleep problems, migraines, joint pain, osteoporosis, osteoarthritis, and eventually kidney failure. Yes, if I had known then what I know now about the alternatives to pain meds, the many direct effects of mixing medications, the countless ways to help with natural sleep and natural detoxing, I may have been able to add more years of a quality life. My wish and I know her wish would have been to help anyone avoid a life of suffering by educating them that they have alternatives to everything. You DO NOT have to accept a diagnosis of doom and gloom from anyone. If you question most and investigate everything your choices will be abundant rather than few. Yes "Knowledge is Power but Action is Influence".

Pass along the information you are about to learn for a tipping is upon us. Change happens when the masses create need. Enjoy and learn!!!

Douglas Caporrino

Introduction

Why am I writing this book and who am I? Let's start with why? There is an amazing amount of misinformation out there today regarding your health, nutrition, supplements and natural cures. There are even more people coming forward claiming to be healers, experts in health, and even medically intuitive. So, what, when and who, do you believe? Tabloids, talk shows and social media outlets talk about "studies" that have been done but no one ever stops to question, who did the studies, who funds the studies, who were the participant's in the study and who stood to gain financially from the study. Yet, news outlets regularly report on the so called "studies" and instill fear into the population. I can't count the number of studies in the last 3 months on whether coffee is good for you or bad for you. Each week a new study comes out negating the study from the week before. I started a company over 14 years ago called Results thru Research, which goes through the most popular health journals and actually breaks down the studies that are most often referred to in the media to see if they are valid and unbiased.

This is why I am writing this book, to help you find the right information on what's best for you or a loved one. I have been researching nutrition and health for the better part of my life. I am now 58 years young and will continue to uncover the real truths behind studies and what's best for all people's health till I no longer can in this lifetime.

Most advertising in the world pertaining to health and nutrition is baseless in its claims which is why the FDA has begun a major crackdown on such advertising. Most if not all ads for drugs start off talking about how wonderful the drug is and what it can prevent and then a picture of a cute little puppy or kitten appears while they go through a lengthy list of side effects or should I say direct effects of that drug, ranging from stroke, heart failure to nothing short of blindness and paralysis. Well just sign me up for that drug.

By the time you finish this book and read it again for a second time you will have a pretty good understanding of what will or won't work for you specifically. You see, my philosophy has always been "we are all biochemically different" so what works for one person may not work for the other when it comes to food and supplements. For one person to come out and say we were all meant to be vegetarians or mixed carnavoirs is as ridiculous as me saying we should all be wearing a size 9 shoe. It just isn't so.

So, who am I and why have I taken on this journey? My name is Douglas Joseph Caporrino and I was born in Hoboken New Jersey. When my mom was in her early 30s she had to go in for an emergency laminectomy surgery under general anesthesia. Unbeknownst to her she found out after the surgery that she was already 3 months pregnant. Doctors told her that she should abort the baby in fear that the surgery may have done harm to the fetus. Refusing to do so she went ahead and had the child, me.

I was born with three holes in my heart, juvenile rheumatoid arthritis and a rare disease called Familial Mediterranean fever. At the time there were only 740 reported cases in the USA. As a child I was prohibited to participate in sports activities in fear that my heart could get worse. I was instructed to not participate in any activities for a few years to see if the holes would start to close if they didn't then open-heart surgery was the next step.

After several years the holes did manage to close and turn to murmurs. At age 11 the handcuffs were taken off and I was free to run and play like a normal child. My arthritis was never really apparent until I started to hit my late teens. As for the rare disease, it was misdiagnosed until I was 18 years of age. For years I would come down with flu like symptoms, loosing vast amounts of weight due to fever and nausea. Doctors would always attribute it to the flu or even possible rheumatic fever. After one severe bout at age 17 that hospitalized me with 106 fever that almost killed me, doctors did a battery of tests. My case was presented to a special infectious disease hospital in NYC and the diagnosis was FMF. The treatment at the time was to put you on a drug called colchicine. The possible side effects of colchicine were: numbness or tingly feeling in your fingers or toes; pale or gray appearance of your lips, tongue, or hands; severe vomiting or diarrhea; easy bruising or bleeding, feeling weak or tired; fever, chills, body aches, flu symptoms.

Well after being on this for about 2 weeks I insisted to be taken off and looked for other methods of controlling or healing this. After meeting a chiropractor/nutritionist in the gym I decided to pursue the holistic approach. I can't say for sure if it were the adjustments, change of diet or just the many supplements I was taking that made the difference but I rarely relapsed for the first year and then almost never after that.

At the age of 18, I decided to compete in an amateur bodybuilding competition the Mr. Teenage New Jersey. After all those years of never being able to work out as a child I found myself a pretty skinny kid in high school, 6'2" 145lbs to be exact so weight lifting became my passion. About 3 weeks out from the competition I was the victim of a hit and run accident as the passenger in a car. Both my knee fat pads were crushed so I needed surgery to repair them so needless to say it knocked me out of my competition. I was determined to come back next year even better and try competing again. I am happy to say that I did and won the show.

Several years later and many shows after I gave up competitive bodybuilding and took up Triathlons. Towards the end of one of training rides on my bicycle I went off the side of a road and into a drainage ditch, head first over the handle bars and landed on a small boulder with my head and shoulder cracking my helmet down the middle. After laying there unconscious, god knows how long, a good samaritan found me and called the paramedics just as I was going into shock. She basically saved my life. I was rushed to the local hospital where I was diagnosed with a fractured shoulder and scapula in many places. Several doctors looked at me and advised against surgery in fear that it was too risky and I could lose use of my left arm completely. A few brave ones said they would attempt it and one confident one, the surgeon for the New York Giants, Dr. Russel Warren from the Hospital for Special Surgery said he has seen this injury before and would fix me. After several hours of surgery, 6 screws, a stainless-steel plate and many bone grafts later, I was put back together. Once again, he never guaranteed me success with the surgery also cautioning me that I may lose motion in my left arm. Well after 4 months I walked back in his office and did a pushup on his floor much to his surprise. He asked what I did to recover and heal so quickly and I replied, I did everything from hyperbaric chamber therapy, to strict nutrition protocols, acupuncture, chiropractic and even live embryotic cell injection from blue sharks. I figured what the heck, maybe it would help swim faster at the very least. LOL I don't know if it was one or a combination of all the things that I did that had a synergistic effect on my healing but I thank the powers that be I am back to running, swimming and biking again and have completed a few Ironman's and many triathlons.

I went to college determined to be a doctor. I did volunteer work at a downtown hospital in NYC while attending school and it gave me a completely different view of what being a doctor was. I decided to pursue biochemistry instead, wowed by the notion that our bodies reacted to physical, chemical and emotional stressors.

While still in school I found myself being a very sought-after personal trainer and became lucky enough to build a large celebrity clientele. I was then asked to be the "Health and Wellness consultant" for the "Joan Rivers Show". That was followed by many of the morning talk and cable shows. Life was good.

I continued my education in the field of nutrition and supplementation and became part of a supplement manufacturing company in Orange County California. I found that many of the larger companies were not using great core ingredients so I went down a path of creating a mostly pure and bio available product line that could be available to the masses.

With the great exposure I had been given I started lecturing on the subject of biochemical differences in each person's body and how we all required different foods. This lead me to traveling up to 20 times a year around the world speaking to audiences as intimate as 20 and as large as 5,000. It also led me into my next company L3W, Live Longer and Live well. With the help of my 2 partners, one a NASA scientist and the other a doctor we created a blood and urine test that was able to determine a person's exact needs for which foods and nutrients they needed. We have seen thousands of patients come through our program with a greater than 80% success rate measured by inflammatory markers in the body.

I now enjoy less travel with the same passion for speaking to large or small crowds and coaching clients from around the world on exactly what foods and supplements they should be incorporating into their life to achieve great health and reverse disease based on specific diagnostic testing. The great thing about this is I do it all via phone.

I continue to compete in triathlons today live the 80/20 rule when it comes to lifestyle.

I would have to say that being born with the challenges that I had led me to the person that I am today.

The companies that I have created have certainly been rewarding but the most rewarding aspects of what I do is my 1 on 1 coaching with the clients from around the world via phone. 9 out of 10 of my clients I have never met but the stories of helping to get someone off several medications, or reversing heart disease in another person or the sound of a mom crying in joy over the phone because her little boy with asthma no longer wheezes makes me tear up in joy.

I look at a person as a whole. What stressors are in their life, both physical, chemical and emotional and address them. I do Micronutrient testing on most of my clients to determine exactly what supplements they need if any. Most disease is caused by deficiencies in the body but until crisis hits we never look for them.

I believe many doctors today are starting to move towards personal medicine like Epigenetics, Immunotherapy for cancers and other great preventative modalities.

This is who I am and why I am writing this book. Congratulations on taking the first step towards a healthier life.

Cancers Many Cures

There is a plethora of so-called natural cures for cancer on the internet these days. An amazing multitude of different cancer cures have been described in books and articles. Former cancer victims have written about their recovery, which often involved nothing more than living peacefully on an organic raw-food diet. Others attribute their cure to immune-enhancing factors, alternative technology or meditation and guided imagery, sometimes to specific remedies, but commonly in various combinations of any of these methods. There are so many combinations and variations; the list seems to be endless.

Doctors and Nutritional Cures

Many years ago, one of the easiest protocols was used by a Danish doctor Kristine Nolfi. She cured her own cancer with a hundred percent organic and vegetarian raw-food diet, and then continued to cure cancer patients in the same way. She lost her medical license for using 'dangerous' and unapproved methods but her fame nevertheless spread throughout Scandinavia.

In New Zealand Dr. Eva Hill did much the same thing to cure her own cancer, and to help many of her patients.

Ann Wigmore pioneered and promoted wheatgrass juice after curing her own cancer with it, in combination with an organic vegetarian diet.

Together with Victoras Kulvinskas she formed the Hippocrates Health Institute in Boston, and branches and health farms using wheatgrass juice quickly sprang up in many countries. It is more effective if a non-centrifugal juicer is used for making juices, or possibly just a mincer with the juice pressed by hand.

In South Africa, Johanna Brand, a Naturopath, invented the now famous grape cure by curing herself of stomach cancer in the 1920's. For six weeks she ate nothing but grapes, black varieties are the best. Thousands of former cancer victims have testified as to the effectiveness of her method. Because it is now so difficult to obtain unsprayed grapes, commercially sprayed grapes have sometimes been used after thorough washing in warm soapy water and careful rinsing.

The Breuss-Cure, which originated in Germany, also lasts for 6 weeks; a maximum of 500 ml of freshly pressed vegetable juices are used, mainly beetroot with some carrot, celery and radish. In addition, herbal teas and onion broth are recommended. It too, is claimed to have cured thousands.

Hans Nieper, a respected German cancer therapist (recently deceased), used in addition to a good diet a wide range of supplements to inhibit tumor growth, activate the immune system, degrade the tumor with large-scale enzyme supplementation, and strengthen the liver and general metabolism. Nieper claimed a 50% survival rate of 'terminal' patients. If patients survive for 18 months on this program, their statistical life expectancy becomes about normal, unlike with chemotherapy where life expectancy continues to drop after 18 months.

Another German cancer therapist, DR J Kuhl, used a diet high in lactic acid fermented foods with good results. Lactic acid produced by a tumor rotates light to the left and enhances tumor growth. Lactic acid produced by lactic acid bacteria, on the other hand, rotates light to the right and inhibits tumor growth.

DR. Johanna Budwig, also in Germany, found high-quality linseed/flax oil combined with 'quark' and a mainly vegetarian raw-food diet most effective. Quark is the German word for cottage cheese, but made from lactic acid fermented raw skim milk as used by Budwig. This provides not only the beneficial fermentation products, but also a high amount of sulfur-amino acids. These are mainly cysteine and methionine, which together with the polyunsaturated fatty acids in linseed/flax oil can quickly restore the oxidative energy production in and around tumors, and cause them to regress.

The Bristol Cancer Help Center in England, formerly under the direction of DR. Alec Forbes, offers a wide-ranging holistic program similar to the Mexican clinics. This includes a vegetarian diet of largely raw foods, supplemented by specific vitamins, minerals, enzymes, ginseng and liver herbs, in addition to colonic cleansing, visualization, biofeedback, relaxation, meditation and spiritual healing.

DR. Maud Fere, in New Zealand, claimed success with a much more limited program that had helped her to cure her own bowel cancer. She advocated a good vegetarian diet, but her main emphasis, similar to Max Gerson's, was that there must be no salt in it. She also found it beneficial to use diluted hydrochloric acid, diluted phosphoric acid, ammonium chloride, and tincture of iodine.

Earlier Are Waerland became famous for a successful diet that consisted of sour milk and similar products, whole grains raw or only partly cooked, as well as fruits and vegetables. There are still many active Waerland groups in Germany and Scandinavia. Bircher-Benner advocated a similar lacto-vegetarian raw-food diet. He invented the by now famous but greatly deteriorated muesli. The macrobiotic diet based on cooked brown rice and only a minimum of raw food is very different from all the other anticancer diets. It has a mild cleansing action and some cancer victims claim to have been cured with a strict macrobiotic diet.

From 1951 DR A. Ferenczi in Hungary used large amounts of beetroot successfully for tumor regression, up to 1 kg daily have been used. The active ingredient is the purple coloring containing anthocyanin. It is now also available as a freeze-dried powder.

The Gerson Therapy

Best known is probably the Gerson therapy. Born in Germany, DR Max Gerson immigrated to the US in 1938. His diet consists mainly of fresh, preferably organic, fruit and vegetables. He stressed a high potassium content that is more in the skins or outer part of root vegetables than in the centers. Sodium, on the other hand, was to be severely restricted - the diet was completely without added salt, but with added potassium salts instead.

In addition, Gerson prescribed hydrochloric acid with pepsin, pancreatin, and high doses of Lugol's solution for iodine together with freeze-dried thyroid, niacin, Royal Jelly and injections of vitamin B12 with crude liver. In addition, raw liver juice was used for its high content of enzymes. Later, with increasing chemicalization of agriculture, the liver juice was omitted while linseed/flax oil was belatedly added to the list of supplements.

Liver detoxification with frequent coffee enemas was another cornerstone of the Gerson Therapy; otherwise patients with advanced cancer might die despite disappearing tumors. Gerson treated hundreds of so-called terminal cases of which about 50 % recovered.

DR Issels used the Gerson therapy successfully in Germany. In addition, he realized the harmful influence of dead or infected teeth and mercury amalgam fillings on the outcome of cancer therapy. Therefore, his patients had to have all unhealthy teeth removed at the beginning of the treatment.

The Kelly approach

DR W. D. Kelly, an American dentist, was given only one month to live with multiple tumors of the liver, pancreas and other organs. He cured himself with a vegetarian raw-food diet with the addition of various supplements, but especially with high doses of pancreatin. Pancreas enzymes are very effective in destroying tumors and sometimes even too effective. Kelly, like Gerson and other holistic cancer therapists, saw the greatest danger in a too rapid destruction of the tumor that can kill the patient with poisons generated by the disintegrating tumor proteins. He recommended daily Epsom salts purges during the critical period and, if required, also coffee enemas.

After helping thousands of patients by supplying individualized information to the patient's doctor, he believes that cancer can usually be cured if there is at least one month, but preferably three months, of life expectancy when starting the program.

As a simple, but somewhat expensive self-test for the early detection of cancer before tumors can be found clinically, he recommends taking six to eight pancreatin tablets after each meal for four weeks. If you feel worse after these four weeks with nausea, headaches or fatigue, there is likely to be a cancerous condition. If you feel better instead, brighter and with more energy, the condition is precancerous. If there is no difference there is probably no early cancer, but there may already be a clinically detectable malignant tumor present.

Kelley has an extensive documentation with 10,000 medically verified diagnoses. In one study all his cases of pancreas cancer were investigated. With conventional treatment there were virtually no survivors after 5 years. He had 22 cases on record. Of these, 10 never started the treatment and survived for 67 days. 7 followed it partially and survived an average of 233 days, while the 5 who followed the Kelley treatment completely all recovered completely.

Aajonus Vonderplanitz, in California, claims great success in overcoming advanced cancer with a raw-food diet that includes raw (organic) meat, see his book We Want to Live (1997).

REMEDIES & HERBS

I recently read that about ten thousand Americans a day cross the border into Mexico for medical treatment. Many of these have US health insurance that is not valid in Mexico. For some the attraction may be cheaper treatment, and for others a more humane face of medicine, but the most important draw card would be the fact that all holistic cancer clinics have effectively been eliminated in the US, and are now just south of the border down Mexico way. While these clinics also give dietary advice, they rely mainly on specific remedies, such as laetrile, ozone therapy, herbs and specific immune enhancing measures, but also visualization and meditation.

Many thousands of former cancer victims have attested to the beneficial effects of laetrile in the treatment of their disease. While not a cure in itself, laetrile has been found in clinical trials to reduce or eliminate cancer-related pain, improve the appetite with weight gain in underweight patients, eliminate the typical nauseating cancer odor in terminal wards and induce a sense of well-being and hope. In animal experiments tumor inhibition was evident. Initially, laetrile commonly is injected, several grams daily, while oral doses of similar amounts may continue for a year or more. Animal experiments showed similar benefits to those from laetrile even when just bitter almonds or apricot kernels were eaten. These are also commonly used in countries where the availability of laetrile is restricted or where its use is illegal.

Garlic is frequently used as a supporting remedy in the treatment of cancer. It has proven anticancer properties. Not only does it protect against the formation of tumors, including metastases, it also inhibits the growth of established tumors. In addition, it strengthens the immune system and improves the detoxifying ability of the liver.

Two other remedies used widely in the Mexican and other cancer clinics are Vitamin C, and hydrazine sulfate. Linus Pauling and Ewan Cameron pioneered Vitamin C treatment for cancer, and found greatly increased survival times for terminal cancer patients with 10 g of Vitamin C daily. Now it is sometimes used in even larger amounts, just below the threshold where it causes diarrhea, initially it may also be infused intravenously.

Hydrazine sulfate was discovered by DR Joseph Gold for use in cancer treatment. It blocks a liver enzyme which converts the lactic acid produced by a tumor back into glucose, a reaction which takes much more energy from the patient than it generates. It was mainly used with 'terminal': patients who reported improved appetite, normalized weight, increased strength and less pain. However, presently it is increasingly used in earlier stages and more and more patients claim that their tumors have disappeared.

Another group of remedies is specifically designed to stimulate the immune system. In the 1950s Krebiozen made headlines in the US, promoted by a respected scientist, DR Andrew Ivy. Five hundred doctors used it, and 20,000 testimonials of cancer victims stood behind DR Ivy and his coworkers at their trial. They were acquitted, but the AMA succeeded in blacklisting Krebiozen.

DR B Coley was an early US cancer pioneer who used a special vaccine to induce fever and inflammation in cancer patients. Out of 500 cases half remained free of malignancy during follow-up for 5-54 years.

Virginia Livingston-Wheeler, an US microbiologist, combined a vegetarian diet with a vaccine prepared from the patient's own body fluids. Most widely used, however, especially in Germany, are vaccines related to the tubercle bacillus that were developed by Prof Enderlein.

In Japan, DR Hasumi claims outstanding success in curing cancer with a vaccine made from the patient's own urine; however, it works only if the immune system is still sufficiently strong.

Somewhat hard to take for many is urine therapy. J W Armstrong in his book The Water of Life relates many cases of medically diagnosed cancer that appeared to be cured after a urine fast usually lasting for about three weeks, drinking nothing but one's own urine and additional water. With this, Armstrong regarded cancer as rather easy to cure; 'child's play' he called it, except if someone had previously already received medical treatment.

The Greek Professor of Internal Medicine, E.V. Danopoulus, discovered that urea was the most potent anticancer factor in urine. At first, he treated several liver cancer patients with it who recovered, and then he also used it successfully with many other advanced cancers. However, after the publication of his results in the Lancet in 1974 he experienced increasing harassment and retired from medical practice.

DR William Lane in the US noticed that sharks do not develop cancer. This prompted him to experiment with good results with shark cartilage that is now commercially available. Liquid bovine cartilage appears now to be preferable to shark cartilage. Also shark oil is useful.

Gaston Naessens in Canada was successful curing cancer by injecting a modified camphor compound into lymph nodes to strengthen the immune system. He claims a long-term remission rate of 75%. His remedy, called 714-X, is now available from Canada and New Zealand.

Thousands of cancer victims, in East European and other poor countries, claim to have been cured by taking refined kerosene. That apparently kills the cancer microbe and possibly cancer cells as well.

DR Seeger, the German cancer researcher, found Zell Oxygen most helpful to 'normalize' cancer cells by restarting their oxidative energy production. Zell Oxygen is a culture of special young yeast cells very high in oxygenating enzymes. It works best combined with Royal Jelly. Wobe-mugos is imported from Germany and contains proteolytic enzymes from hydrolyzed beef pancreas, thymus and other glands. It is claimed to be very beneficial in so-called terminal conditions.

Herbal Remedies

Essiac (Ojibway Indian Tea) is another famous cancer herb mixture developed about 1922 by the Canadian nurse Rene Caisse. In 1937 the Royal Cancer Commission found that Essiac was effective against cancer and in 1938 Essiac came within three votes of being legalized as a remedy for terminal cancer. After this, Rene received special permission to treat terminal cancer patients but was not allowed to take money for it. At the time of her death in 1978 the Canadian Ministry of Health & Welfare destroyed her huge collection of documents and patient files on the effectiveness of Essiac.

The four ingredients are rhubarb root, burdock root and slippery elm as blood purifiers and the tops of young sheep's sorrel (Rumen acetosella) to destroy cancer cells. The use of Essiac is gradually spreading to other countries but there is also a warning that some distributors have substituted yellow dock or curly dock for the essential sheep's sorrel.

A tea made from leaves and stems or twigs of papaw is another traditional cancer remedy. It was revealed to Stan Sheldon on the Queensland Gold Coast in 1962, who cured his rapidly spreading tumors in both lungs within two months. This remedy is now widely used throughout Queensland. According to an article in New Scientist, a chemical has been discovered in one kind of papaw, which is one billion times more effective against cancer cells than presently used anticancer drugs. An Aboriginal cancer remedy is the maroon bush, while the use of mistletoe preparations is based on ancient European folklore and recommendations by Rudolf Steiner.

Jethro Kloss was a well-known early American herbalist of the 'old school'. For cancer treatment he used mainly red clover blossoms, violet leaves and flowers, the roots of burdock and yellow dock, golden seal, echinachea, aloes, agrimony, dandelion root, supposedly with good success.

Even more famous and most widely used in many countries, is the Hoxsey herb mixture. It originated about 1925 in the US with thousands of patients attesting to its usefulness in overcoming their cancer. The internal remedy consists of amarga, berberis root, buckthorn bark, burdock, licorice, pokeroot, prickly ash, red clover, stillingia root and potassium iodide. There were also three external remedies to be painted on any visible tumors to make them dry up and fall out. Presently mainly Herbveil 8 and KC101 (in NZ) and cansema are being used for melanoma and other skin cancers as well as tumors close to the skin, such as breast tumors.

Jason Winters described his own cure from terminal cancer in his book 'Killing Cancer'. In addition to diet, he used red clover, chaparral, gotu kola, selenium and some not well-defined roots and spices in his herb mixture, which is not available in most countries.

ALTERNATIVE TECHNOLOGY

Ozone therapy has been pioneered in Germany, and it is used there as well as in the Mexican cancer clinics by thousands of doctors, not only for treating cancer, but also AIDS, and other serious infectious diseases. Generally, about 220 ml of the patient's blood is mixed with ozone, often under pressure, and then re-injected into a vein. This kills not only cancer cells and the cancer microbe in the treated blood but in the whole body, while the immune system is strengthened at the same time. Where ozone therapy is not available, patients commonly take diluted hydrogen peroxide.

A similar beneficial effect is achieved with overheating a tumor. Cancer cells are damaged or weakened by temperatures of 42-43C, which are still harmless for normal cells. To overheat internal tumors, daily bath temperatures are gradually raised over a period of weeks or months up to 47C. Various precautions are required, especially the blood sugar level needs to be kept artificially low during treatment; otherwise tumor growth may be stimulated if temperatures are not quite high enough. As after ozone therapy, the damaged tumor becomes highly responsive to any additional holistic therapy. In addition, the blood circulation is greatly increased.

The south-pointing pole of a magnet inhibits not only microbes but also cancer cells. Tumors could be inhibited or regressed by long exposure to a strong south-pointing pole of 4000 gauss or more. This also appears to reduce pain, inflammation and infections. Presently many cancer patients use electronic zappers and magnetic pulsars with apparently good success. The most commonly used varieties are the Hulda Clark zapper and the Beck zapper or blood purifier, recommended to be used in combination with oxygen therapy and colloidal silver.

Similar results may be achieved by radiating the tumor site with strong blue light. An article in New Scientist revealed that blue light inhibits cell divisions; it is also used in some hospitals as the quickest cure for jaundiced babies.

The Tronado machine is a German invention to shine very high radio frequencies onto a tumor area. It overheats the tumor and causes its destruction but unlike conventional radiotherapy, it does not damage the surrounding healthy tissue.

DR John Holt, a radio-therapist at the Sir Charles Gairdner Hospital in Perth, managed with the help of the then Premier of Western Australia, John Tonkin, to buy a Tronado for the hospital, and in addition, one for his private clinic. Holt treated more than seven thousand cancer patients with the Tronado with remarkable results. At the same time, he continued to treat cancer patients at the hospital with normal radiotherapy.

In a published trial with head and neck cancers (for easy verification of results) a 34 % initial success rate was achieved with radiotherapy while after three years 17 % were still in remission. With the Tronado the initial success was 92 % and after three years 68 %. However, such are the mysterious ways of the medical profession that only the Tronado in private practice could be used, until quite recently the one installed at the hospital was never allowed to be operated.

The Roy Ray Rife electronic frequency instrument emitted waves of a frequency that was specific to kill cancer cells. Conventional research institutions confirmed a high success rate before the AMA (US) took court action and destroyed the treatment machines. Now there are replicas appearing, some of which seem to be more effective than others.

The US magazine The Choice (Spring 1990) published an article about Nick van Echteld, who claims to have completely recovered from terminal metastatic cancer in 1989. Echteld attributes his remarkable cure to self-treatment with a Rife instrument, while his orthodox specialists believe instead in 'spontaneous remission' - a cure without cause.

Wilhelm Reich attributed his success with terminal cancer patients to their immersion in a strong field of bio-energy or orgone, as he called it. Orgone accumulators are easy to build with alternating layers of metal and organic material. More recently 'orgonite' is being used, a mixture of a resin with fine metal particles.

Harold S Burr discovered the electric life fields around living organisms. Tumors have an abnormal negative charge as compared to the surrounding healthy tissue. In Sweden Bjorn Nordenstrom used 10-volt needle-like electrodes inserted into a tumor to destroy it. For external tumors, I experimented with a large flat 1.5-volt positive electrode on the tumor and the negative electrode on a healthy tissue nearby.

Finally, I may mention that various cancer victims claim to have been cured by psychic surgery, especially in the Philippines. Also, radionic instruments are sometimes claimed to be successful with cancer.

MIND IMPROVEMENT

Wilhelm Reich discovered the harmful effects of repressed sexual feelings in the development of cancer. His methods for freeing up feelings and energy flows have become standard practice in bio-energy therapy and other holistic treatments.

Another ten-year study published in the Lancet, of women with advanced metastatic breast cancer found that just belonging to a support group and meeting once a week, doubled the life span as compared to a control group that had medically been treated in the same way. In addition to some well-known support groups, such as those run by the Bristol clinic in England, or Ian Gawler's support group in Victoria (Australia), there are now small groups, often in connection with meditation groups, in many cities.

Well known for his meditation work with cancer patients was DR A Meares of Melbourne. In the US the Simontons have pioneered guided imagery in cancer treatment. They showed that survival times with terminal cancers can be doubled in this way. Characteristics in patients, which they found to be associated with above average results are emotional resilience, flexible beliefs, physical activity, strong self-concept and social autonomy. Many cancer patients have been greatly helped and seem to have recovered mainly because they learned to express their feelings and emotions and they moved towards fulfilling their emotional needs.

Of all the published, properly randomized clinical trials, psychotherapy is by far the most effective cancer therapy. Eysenk and Grossarth-Maticek (Behavior Research and Therapy 1991; 29 (1):17-31) found that 13 years after extended individual therapy none of 50 patients in the treated cancer-prone group had died but 32 percent in the control group. With group therapy, after 7 years, there were 18 out of 239 cancer death in the treated group, compared to 111 of the 234 in the control group. With terminal cancer patients the increased survival time was 64% and women with metastasized breast cancer lived about twice as long.

The most powerful setback to recovery, on the other hand, is a medical pronouncement that the condition in incurable and terminal, especially if a time limit is mentioned. This then becomes a self-fulfilling hypnotic suggestion; just like "pointing the bone" in other cultures and it is then difficult for a holistic therapist to change this medically implanted death wish into hope and faith that are the keys for recovery.

The most promising therapy appears to be The New Medicine of the much-persecuted German DR Hamer. He claims a 95% success rate by discovering and eliminating the emotional shock that triggered the development of cancer, commonly one to two years before its diagnosis. My own preference is a combination of DR Hamer's approach, with an organic raw-food diet that is suitable for the metabolic type of the patient.

Cancer Treatments True Hero

Alternative cancer treatments are a kind of "forbidden area" in medicine, but Dr. Gonzalez chose to go that route anyway, and has some remarkable success stories to show for his pioneering work. His passing in July of 2015 was one of the great loses to the healing world.

He didn't set out to treat cancer at first however, let alone treat patients. His original plan was to be a basic science researcher at Sloan-Kettering, a teaching hospital for Cornell Medical College. He had a chance meeting with William Kelley, a controversial dentist who was one of the founders of nutritional typing. Dr. Kelley had been practicing alternative- and nutritional approaches for over two decades at the time, led him to begin a student project investigation of Kelley's work, in the summer of 1981.

"I started going through his records and even though I was just a second year medical student, I could see right away there were cases that were extraordinary," he says. *"Patients with appropriately diagnosed pancreatic cancer, metastatic breast cancer in the bone, metastatic colorectal cancer… who were alive 5, 10, 15 years later under Kelley's care with a nutritional approach."*

This preliminary review led to a formal research study, which Dr. Gonzalez completed while doing his fellowship in cancer, immunology and bone marrow transplantation.

The "Impossible" Recoveries of Dr. Kelley's Cancer Patients

After going through thousands of Kelley's records, Dr. Gonzalez put together a monograph, divided into three sections:

- Kelley's theory
- 50 cases of appropriately-diagnosed lethal cancer patients still alive five to 15 years after diagnosis, whose long-term survival was attributed to Kelley's program
- Patients Kelley had treated with pancreatic cancer between the years 1974 and 1982

According to Dr. Good, the president of Sloan-Kettering who had become Gonzalez' mentor, if Kelley could produce even one patient with appropriately diagnosed pancreatic cancer who was alive 5-10 years later, it would be remarkable. They ultimately tracked down 22 of Kelley's cases.

Ten of them met him once and didn't do the program after being dissuaded by family members or doctors who thought Kelley was a quack.

The average survival for that group was about 60 days.

A second group of seven patients who did the therapy partially and incompletely (again, dissuaded by well-intentioned but misguided family members or doctors), had an average survival of 300 days.

The third group consisting of five patients, who were appropriately diagnosed with advanced pancreatic cancer and who completed the full program, had an average survival of **eight and a half years!** In Dr. Gonzalez' words, this was "just unheard of in medicine."

One of those patients included a woman diagnosed by the Mayo Clinic with stage four pancreatic cancer who had been given six months to live. She'd learned about Kelley's program through a local health food store. She completed his treatment and is still alive today, 29 years later.

The Truth about Medical Journals: Why Gonzalez's Book Was Never Published

However, despite—or rather *because of*—the remarkable success of the treatment, Gonzalez couldn't get his findings published.

"We tried to publish case reports in the medical journals; the whole book, parts of the book, individual case reports—with no success," he says.

This is an important point that many fail to realize.

Those of us who practice natural medicine are frequently criticized for not publishing our findings. My justification for that is that it's not going to be published anyway, and Dr. Gonzalez' anecdotal story confirms this view.

His mentor and supporter, Dr. Good, was one of the most published authors in the scientific literature at that point, with over 2,000 scientific articles to his name. He'd been nominated for the Nobel Prize three times, and yet he was refused because the findings were "too controversial," and flew in the face of conventional medical doctrine.

If the cream of the crop is refused, how does a general primary care physician get an article published?

He doesn't...

"Robert Good was at the top of his profession: President of Sloan-Kettering, father of modern immunology, and did the first bone marrow transplant in history. Yet, he couldn't get it published," Gonzalez says. *"He couldn't even get a single case report published.*

In fact, I have a letter from one of the editors, dated 1987, who wrote a blistering letter to Good saying "You've been boondoggled by a crazy quack guy. Don't you see this is all a fraud?"

It was just the most extraordinary, irrational letter... [Because] the patients' names were there, the copies of their pertinent medical records were there... Any of them could have called these patients, like Arlene Van Straten who, 29 years later, will talk to anyone... But no one cared. They wouldn't do it; they didn't believe it.

They couldn't believe *it.*

It was very disturbing to me because I say, "It is what it is." I come out of a very conventional research orientation, and it was astonishing to me—I had assistance; I had the president of Sloane-Kettering who couldn't get this thing published because it disagreed with the philosophy that was being promoted in medicine; that only chemotherapy, radiation, or immunotherapy can successfully treat cancer, even though the success rate was abysmal.

The idea that medical journals are these objective and unbiased repositories of the truths about science is total nonsense. Most of them are owned by the drug companies. They won't publish anything that disagrees with their philosophy."

By the end of 1987, it was clear that the work would never get published, and since Dr. Good had retired from Sloan-Kettering, they no longer had the power-base to conduct clinical trials.

Dr. Kelley, realizing his work would never be accepted, let alone get published, "went off the deep end," in Dr. Gonzalez' words, and stopped seeing patients altogether. Dr. Gonzalez self-published the Kelley cases in 2010 in his book **One Man Alone** (Available on Amazon). In his lifetime, he wrote four books which you can see here at **www.newspringpress.com**. In fact, he wrote a book entitled **What Went Wrong** about the NCI clinical trial that was sabotaged.

"When I last spoke to him in the summer of 1987, he accused me of being part of a CIA plot to steal his work, and I knew that I had to move on," Dr. Gonzalez says.

"To this day, of course, I give him credit for his brilliant innovation. It's kind of like Semmelweis, who ended up going crazy during the 19th century after showing doctors should wash their hands before delivering babies and no one accepted that. Semmelweis just went off the deep end, and that's what kind of what happened to Kelley, I say with great sadness."

Starting the Alternative Cancer Treatment Practice

Dr. Gonzalez set up a practice in New York together with his colleague, Dr. Linda Isaacs, and started seeing patients using Kelley's three-pronged approach. The results were impressive.

One of his remarkable success stories includes a woman diagnosed with inflammatory breast cancer, which is the most aggressive form. She'd been given a death sentence.

Today, over 23 years later, she's still alive and well, and cancer free.

"Here's a woman that was given six months to a year to live AND developed metastases while getting aggressive multi-agent chemotherapy, yet 23 and a half years later, she's alive and well, enjoying her life and just doing so well.

We could see that Kelley's approach really worked and when I report these cases I'm giving Kelley the credit because he developed this treatment," Dr. Gonzalez says.

Recognition from the National Cancer Institute

In 1993, as part of a legitimate effort to reach out to alternative practitioners, the National Cancer Institute (NCI) invited Dr. Gonzalez to present 25 of his cases in a closed-door, invitation-only session. On the basis of that presentation, the NCI suggested he conduct a pilot study with patients diagnosed with advanced pancreatic cancer, which in conventional medicine is known to be an untreatable, highly lethal form of cancer.

Interestingly, Nestle stepped in to finance this pilot study. It may seem an odd choice, but the business motivation was the same then as it is today—making junk food appear healthier is a good business move, even if it's only in theory.

Supervised directly by Dr. Ernst Wynder, a premier cancer researcher, the study was completed in early 1999 and published in June that year. According to Dr. Gonzalez:

"It showed the best results for the treatment of pancreatic cancer in the history of medicine."

Chemo Therapy vs. the Kelley Treatment

To put his results in perspective, the chemo drug, Gemzar, approved for pancreatic cancer dates back to 1997, and the major study that led to its approval had 126 patients. Of those, 18 percent lived one year. Not a single patient out of the 126 lived beyond 19 months.

Dr. Gonzalez' study had 11 participants, of which:

- Five survived for two years
- Four survived three years
- Two survived five years

Based on these results, the NCI decided to fund a large scale clinical trial, to the tune of $1.4 million, to test his nutritional approach against the best chemo available at the time.

"My friends say "Why did you get involved with something like this? How could you trust the NCI?"

Well, the NCI had been very fair, up to that point, and the then-director, Richard Klausner, in face-to-face meetings with him said he thought I was doing something really interesting and needed to be properly supported," Dr. Gonzalez says.

But that goodwill soon disappeared.

How to Sabotage a Clinical Study 101

About a year after the study was approved, Klausner left the NCI and was replaced by new management with a wholly different attitude.

"[F]rom our first meeting, we knew something has changed significantly," Dr. Gonzalez says, *"and all the people that had initially been assigned to the*

study, who were supportive and believed we were doing something useful, were taken off it. In fact, one of them couldn't even talk to me. She said she'd be fired if she talked to me; if she took my phone call.

I was told by another person who had supported me at the NIH that I shouldn't call him at his office; that he was afraid his line was tapped, and I should only call him at home.

That's how insane the politics over this clinical study got. I couldn't believe it! I thought this was just something you'd read about or see on TV, or that some paranoid or crazy person would make up. But here I was living it. Coming out of Robert Good's group, I don't say that to impress people, but my background is so pure and conventional! It was unbelievable to see that the profession I respected and wanted to join could behave like this."

Unfortunately, the study was, in the end, sabotaged.

"Turned out the principal investigator at Columbia, who's supposed to be completely neutral, had helped develop a chemo regimen that was being used against us—a conflict of interest that was never declared," Dr. Gonzalez explains.

"[T]here are specific requirements for entry into a clinical study. Ours is a nutritional program, and when the first protocol version was written, we had a list of specified criteria... They have to be able to eat...Ours is a nutritional program, so patients have to be able to eat. If they can't eat, they can't do the therapy. They have to be able to take care of themselves...

This is a program the patients have to follow at home.

... Initially, the patients could do it and responded to the treatment. Then, there was a sudden change, around 2000-2001, when the Columbia group took total control of the entry of patients in the study. We were excluded from that process, except during the initial months. The thinking was that if we were involved in the admission process, we'd enter the dreaded bias, whereas if conventional doctors were in control, they couldn't possibly be biased.

Of course, the chief investigator helped develop the chemo regimen used in the study. That's virtually the definition of a 'potential bias'!

He started sending us patients that couldn't eat. We had patients that were so sick we would never have accepted them into our private practice. That were so sick, they died before they got the treatment.

Whether it was a trick to the protocol or not, the Columbia team, the NCI, and the NHI insisted that we had an "intent to treat provision into protocol". This means that the minute a patient is accepted into the trial, they're considered treated, even if they never do the therapy. So, the chief of the study at Columbia would enter patients that were so sick, several died before they could pursue their treatment. But because of this intent to treat provision into protocol, they were considered treatment failures.

Ultimately, 39 patients were entered for treatment. Maybe at best, being kind and optimistic, maybe five or six actually did it, the great majority were so sick they couldn't do it."

As a result, the chemo treatment appeared to be a clear winner in this head-to-head evaluation of treatments against incurable pancreatic cancer.

In 2006, Dr. Gonzalez and his partner filed a complaint with the Office of the Human Research Protection (OHRP), which is a group responsible for making sure federal-funded clinical trials are run properly. After a two-year investigation, the OHRP determined that 42 out of 62 patients had been admitted inappropriately. Unfortunately, this never made it to the media, and the Columbia team was able to publish the research findings without mentioning the results of the OHRP review.

Gonzalez's Three-Pronged Approach to Cancer Treatment

Although most of the studies done on this approach were done on pancreatic cancer, Dr. Gonzalez uses it to treat ALL cancers, from brain cancer to leukemia. His treatment, which is based on Kelley's work, consists of three protocols: diet, supplements and enzymes, and detoxification.

The Dietary Protocol:

The cornerstone of the treatment is a personalized diet based on your nutritional- or metabolic type.

Dr. Kelley originally had 10 basic diets and 90 variations that ranged from pure vegetarian and raw food, to heavy-protein meals that included red meat three times a day.

"In terms of diet, Kelley... found that patients diagnosed with the typical solid tumors: tumors of the breast, lungs, stomach, pancreas, liver, colon, uterus, ovaries, and prostate needed a more vegetarian diet," Dr. Gonzalez explains. *"But he had all gradations of a vegetarian diet; one that was 80 percent raw, one that was 80 percent cooked. So even on the vegetarian side, there were all different variations.*

Some had minimal animal protein, some had fish, some had also red meat.

A patient with immune cancer (leukemia, lymphoma, myeloma, and sarcomas, (which are connective tissue cancers that are related to immune cancers) tended to do best on a high-fat, high meat diet.

... Then there are balanced people that do well with a variety of foods, both plant foods and animal products, but they don't tend to get cancer.

Cancer tends to occur on the extremes, the extreme vegetarians—those that tend to be too acid—or extreme meat eaters, who tend to be too alkaline. Balanced people don't tend to get cancer too much. So, we continued the individualized approach, as did Kelley."

Individualized Supplementation and Enzyme Protocol:

The second component is an individualized supplement protocol, designed for your particular metabolism.

"For example, our vegetarian patients need completely different supplements from our meat eaters. The vegetarians do very well with most of the B vitamins, while the meat eaters don't. The vegetarians don't do well with vitamin A, but the meat eaters do. The vegetarians do well with vitamin D; the meat eaters not so well with large doses, and so on," Dr. Gonzalez explains.

"The meat eaters do well with calcium ascorbate as a vitamin C source, while the vegetarians do well with large doses of ascorbic acid. So, the supplement protocols are very individualized and very precisely engineered."

Omega-3 fats are also prescribed, but even here Dr. Gonzalez prescribes different types of omega-3's depending on the patient's nutritional type. In his experience, vegetarians, or carbohydrate types, tend to fare better on flaxseed oil, which contains alpha linoleic acid (ALA) – a plant-based omega 3.

"It is thought that the conversion of the plant-based ALA into the fish-oil based eicosapentaenoic acid (EPA) and docosahexaenoic acid (DHA) is not that efficient," he says, *"But we find that our vegetarian patients actually do it very well and don't use the fish oil or animal-based omega-3 fatty acids as effectively."*

Chia and hemp seed oils can also be used.

Protein types, on the other hand, appear to need the EPA and the DHA and do better on animal-based omega-3 such as krill oil.

"They don't do well with flaxseed," he says. *"Those are the people who can't make the conversion."*

In addition to vitamins, minerals and trace elements, he also prescribes large doses of pancreatic enzymes.

"The essence of Kelley's work was based on the work of Dr. Beard, which goes back to the turn of the last century, about 110 years ago. Beard was a professor at the University of Edinburg, an embryologist actually, not a medical researcher, who first proposed that pancreatic proteolytic enzymes are the main defense against cancer in the body and are useful as a cancer treatment," he explains.

When treating cancer, however, he found it's important to take the right ratio of active and inactive enzymes. The *inactive precursors* are particularly active against cancer. They also have far longer shelf life, and are more stable.

"That would be my advice – get an enzyme that isn't completely activated," Dr. Gonzalez says. *"More active isn't better when it comes to pancreatic enzymes, just like more and more D isn't better than getting the right dosage. You want the right proportions of activated and inactive—most of it as an inactive precursor."*

His proprietary enzyme formula is manufactured by NutriCology. According to Dr. Gonzalez, pancreatic enzymes are not only useful as treatment for active cancer but are also one of the best preventive measures.

Antioxidants, such as astaxanthin, are also very helpful, both in the prevention and treatment of cancer.

The Detoxification Protocol:

The third component is a detoxification routine. Coffee enemas are used to help your liver and kidneys to mobilize and eliminate dead cancer cells that have been broken down by the pancreatic enzymes.

Coffee enemas, although often scoffed at today, were actually used as part of conventional medicine all the way up to the 1960s, and were included in the Merck Manual, which was a handbook for conventional medical treatments into the 1970s.

"They fell out of favor not because they didn't work, but because the drug industry took over medicine, so things like coffee enemas were kind of laughed at," Dr. Gonzalez says. *"So, Kelley learned about coffee enemas from conventional literature and incorporated them into his program and found them extremely helpful."*

When you drink coffee, it tends to suppress your liver function, but when taken rectally as an enema, the caffeine stimulates nerves in your lower bowels, which causes your liver to release toxins as a reflex. Other detox strategies include colon cleanses and liver flushes developed by Kelley.

It's important to realize, however, that **conventional coffee should NOT be used for enemas. The coffee MUST be organic**, naturally caffeinated coffee, and were you to do this at home, you'd also want to use non-bleached filters to avoid introducing toxins into your colon.

"[Organic coffee] is loaded with antioxidants," Dr. Gonzalez says. *"In fact, there are recent studies showing that coffee loaded with antioxidants can have an anti-cancer effect and that coffee may actually help suppress cancer.*

But you have to use organic coffee, it has to have caffeine, and you have to use a coffee maker that doesn't have aluminum, and preferably no plastic."

Dr. Gonzalez also relies on sodium alginate as a detoxifying agent.

"We have a preparation that we put together and it's very effective... It's an algae and it chelates heavy metals and halides. I never use intravenous chelation; we just use sodium alginate."

He recommends taking three capsules three times a day, away from meals, for six weeks to detoxify your body of heavy metals, such as mercury, and halides.

For more information about Dr. Gonzalez and his legacy, visit **www.thegonzalezprotocol.com**. His wife has since published three new books that he was working on before his death called **Conquering Cancer- Volumes 1 & 2- a total of 112 Cancer Patients on the Gonzalez ProtocolÒ** (Available on Amazon) and lastly **Nutrition and The Autonomic Nervous System: The Scientific Foundations of the Gonzalez ProtocolÒ.** Also, due out in 2019 will be one more work called **Proof of Concept** that will include the 25 cases that Dr. Gonzalez presented to the NCI.

In an age of cut, burn and poison cancer, these are just a few options that have been experimented with around the world. I am not recommending one or the other or one over the other, I am merely laying out options that many people have successfully pursued.

The Paleo Diet

Diets come, and diets go. And like fashion, if you wait long enough, what is now out will eventually return – remember almost all information is not new just re-packaged. And when you think about it, that only makes sense. After all, food really falls into one of only three groups: proteins, fats, and carbohydrates. So, all diets are pretty much restricted to mixing things up within those three groups. Ahh, but given those limitations, there is still infinite variety — thus the ever-new diet programs.

And now it is the turn of the Paleo Diet (also known as the Paleolithic Diet, or Caveman Diet) to sweep the nation. In fact, RTR has been literally bombarded with requests for me to explore the topic over the last several months. But in truth, it's not actually new. It was first popularized by Walter Voegtlin in the 1970's and is close cousin to the Atkins diet and the Meat Lovers Diets that rose to popularity about ten years ago with that in mind, let's take a look at the Paleo Diet.

The theory behind the Paleo Diet

As I mentioned, the Paleo Diet has its roots in Walter Voegtlin's book, The Stone Age Diet, which was published in the mid 70's. Originally, it was referred to as the caveman diet, or the stone age diet. "Paleolithic," by the way, is just the scientific term for "old stone age." The theory is that without access to modern diets, cavemen ate more naturally than we do today. They didn't eat Twinkies® and chips and Big Macs®. They were hunter-gatherers and ate as the human body was designed to eat… theoretically. They had no agriculture, no storage facilities, no grocery stores, and no processed foods. They ate wild plants and fresh meat as they found it.

And they were healthy…again, so the theory goes. There was no arthritis, no cancer, no osteoporosis, and no heart disease. They were strong-boned, hearty and healthy, and if they died young, it was not because of disease but because of accidents and a hard environment. And although there are few remains of cavemen to verify the claims, there are a couple of small studies that do indeed show health benefits for those who follow the diet. But mostly there are testimonials. Now please understand, I do not make light of testimonials. I find them potentially as valid as many so-called scientific studies. However, I am quite aware of how testimonials can be ruled by emotion and run totally out of control, totally invalidating themselves. Another problem is that when giving testimonials, people tend to generalize their experiences — if I feel better because of it, then everyone in the world will feel better. That said, the primary argument on behalf of the Paleo Diet is that there are select populations living in the world today that have followed the Paleolithic diet for generations and show none of the signs of modern disease…maybe.

For about 30 years, the Paleo Diet struggled along, taking a back seat to the Atkins Diet®, the Blood Type Diet, the Nutritional Type Diet, Jenny Craig®, Nutrisystem®, the Hollywood Diet®, Volumetrics®, the Mediterranean Diet, the South Beach Diet®, the Carb Lovers Diet, and on and on. It was not until 2005 that the Paleo Diet came into its own, with the publication of Loren Cordain's *The Paleo Diet for Athletes: A Nutritional Formula for Peak Athletic Performance.* With athletes beginning to endorse the diet, it gained momentum, hitting the big time in 2010, with the publication of Cordain's next book, *The Paleo Diet* and Rob Wolf's book, *The Paleo Solution.*

So, what exactly does the Paleo Diet advocate, and is it as good as claimed?

The tenets of the Paleo Diet

The primary tenet of the Paleo Diet is that diets and health started to go downhill the moment agriculture started to gain traction. Farming, the foods it produces, and food processing — which are the cornerstones of the modern diet — are the enemies of health. If you want to be healthy, you have to eat the diet your body was designed for — the diet that cavemen ate, the diet that is natural to man

To summarize, the Paleo Diet is based on what we "think" cavemen ate, based on some historical data and studies of modern-day hunter-gatherers, as well as trace evidence found in archeological digs and a whole lot of guess work and theory. And since true caveman foods are no longer available to us, it is also based on modern food "equivalents" that have been refined over centuries and that are commonly available in today's supermarkets. That means that, for the most part, the meat you eat comes from domesticated animals raised using modern mass production methods, even if grass-fed, and the so called "forage" that you eat is based on cultivated hybrids nurtured on artificial fertilizers and possibly pesticides.

But that's only part of the story. The Paleo Diet is defined as much by what you cannot eat, as by what you can eat. Or more specifically, the philosophy behind the diet is that you are only allowed to eat what was "natural" to the human diet during the Paleolithic era, not the "artificial" foods that have been added to the diet since then as a result of the agricultural revolution and the introduction of urbanization and mass manufacturing. That means that all crops that only became viable parts of the diet because of the agricultural revolution (grains, beans, and peanuts, for example) and the byproducts of domesticated livestock (i.e., dairy) are taboo. Sugar is not allowed. And alcoholic beverages and fermented foods are also off the table.

I think it's pretty much safe to say that if Paleolithic men and women abstained from alcohol, they would have been pretty much alone in the practice — which brings up an interesting contradiction in the Paleolithic diet. If cave-people ate fermented foods, and yet you choose to exclude those foods from the Paleo Diet, which is supposed to be based on what they ate, then you've opened up a fundamental hole in the logic behind the diet. But there's no need to dwell on that now.

One problem we face when looking at the Paleo Diet is that there are multiple versions of it among its many adherents. For example, some insist on organic, grass-fed beef, others barely mention it. Some say no oils are allowed. Others say low omega 6/high omega 3 oils such as canola oil are okay. And others disagree as to which fruits and vegetables are allowed. This brings up a second fundamental problem when discussing the Paleo Diet, with so many variations, what exactly is it? But in general, here is a list of the do's and don'ts of the Paleo Diet.

No grains, beans, potatoes, or dairy

This is numero uno! As the theory goes, for millions of years, humans and their relatives ate meat, fish, poultry, and the leaves, roots, and fruits of many plants. That was their natural diet, and that was their sole diet. Grains, beans, and potatoes were not eaten because uncooked, they are inedible — in fact, according to the theory, they are toxic if eaten raw. (We'll get back to this later, because it's actually not quite true.)

Around 10,000 years ago, two things happened that changed the way we eat. First, humans learned that they could eat the three demon foods — grains, beans, and potatoes — as long as they are thoroughly cooked. Cooking destroys "most" of the toxins that made them inedible. "Most" is the important word here for Paleo's. In any event, these discoveries changed the course of history. No longer did people have to chase animals across the plains and scavenge for roots and berries in harsh winter landscapes. Now they could grow food, store it in granaries for times of famine, and have a source of abundant calories in a stable environment. In addition, they could start raising herds of animals and introduce dairy products into the diet. Once the hunt for food was no longer the driving factor in life, people could devote themselves to the things that make for civilization: This is the point in history that divides Paleolithic man from modern man (or so the theory goes).

Unfortunately, according to the Paleo diet, our bodies are not designed to handle these "new foods." We're not genetically equipped to handle a diet heavy in grains, legumes, and potatoes. And the development of the culinary arts has only exacerbated the problem by introducing salt and sugar to our diets. And now, with the introduction of artificial flavors and colors, preservatives, pesticides, it is more than our bodies can handle. Chronic illness and obesity is the inevitable result.

So, what do grains, beans, potatoes, and dairy have in common that makes them so unhealthy that we have been unable to adapt to them over the last 10,000 years? Two things according to the theory: enzyme blockers and lectins. Plants use enzyme blockers to stop plant seeds from sprouting prematurely. And lectins are natural pesticides used by plants to defend against bacteria, insects, worms, rodents, and other pests that threaten their existence. And when you think about it, from the plants', humans are just another pest that threatens their existence — and thus lectins, defend against people too. Theoretically then, plant lectins are harmful to people. As for dairy, milk contains lectins because the cows eat foods that contain them — and so they are passed on in the milk. I know that the Paleo banishing of milk will certainly draw the attention of the raw milk aficionados who regularly write into the Foundation professing the virtues of raw milk — most of which I acknowledge. But I find that complaint secondary to the fact that lectins are present in meat for the same reason they're present in dairy — because the cattle eat them as part of their diet. So, if you can't have dairy for that reason, how does meat get a free pass? In any case, this argument is somewhat curious since every living thing has defense mechanisms to protect itself from being devoured by predators large and small. For example, humans have immune systems (and antibiotics of their own creation) to defend against bacteria. How can anything "eat" those defenses, figuratively speaking? Because, quite simply, species are constantly adapting to be able to overcome other species' defenses and so use them for food. It is the way of life. But let's not dwell on the negatives; let's move on.

Since lectins are so fundamental to the Paleo Diet, let's explore them in a little more detail. Incidentally, this is not the first time I've explored lectins in some detail

Lectins

Lectins are carbohydrate-binding proteins that are found in most plants, particularly grains, potatoes, and beans. The problem is that some lectins ape the glycoproteins on red blood cells, thus triggering immune reactions in sensitive individuals. And yes, there is no question that different foods definitely have high allergy potential for many people, but the problem appears to be less with the lectins, than with the ability of the digestive tract to fully break down the proteins in the food. And beyond that, lectins are not exclusive to plants. All foods contain lectins. Not all are harmful. Some are actually beneficial. In animals, lectins serve a number of biological functions, from the control of protein levels in the blood to removing harmful glycoproteins from the circulatory system to recognizing carbohydrates that are found exclusively on certain pathogens and thus targeting them for elimination.

For example, guava lectin may be useful in the prevention of E. coli infection of the gut._Even better, some studies have shown that lectins can neutralize cancer cells. Soy and peanut lectins appear to be particularly good in this regard.

But not all lectins are good. Curiously, soy and peanut lectins, which may target cancer cells, are also among the most allergenic lectins in nature. One lectin with an especially bad rep and in the news over the last few years is gluten. Like most lectins, gluten is resistant to stomach acid and digestive enzymes and does not break down easily in the gut. Once in the gut, it may attach to the intestinal wall and damage its lining. Gluten has been implicated in a whole range of intestinal diseases such as irritable bowel syndrome, colitis, Crohn's, and of course, Celiac-Sprue. More specifically, gluten, in those susceptible, can break down the surface of the small intestine, stripping it of mucus and causing the gut to leak — allowing undigested proteins to pass into the bloodstream.

According to some proponents of the Paleo Diet, lectins may also play a role in diabetes by tricking cells into thinking they've been stimulated by insulin and also by causing the beta cells of the pancreas to release insulin. Yet other lectins may play a role in rheumatoid arthritis by attaching to cell surfaces and tricking the immune system into thinking that cells are actually pathogens, thus triggering the immune system to attack the body — an autoimmune response. And to be sure, there is no question that certain foods definitely have high allergy potential for many people, but the problem appears to be less with the lectins, than with the ability of the digestive tract to fully break down the proteins in the food. As I've discussed many times before, the use of digestive enzymes with meals and proteolytic enzymes between meals can often help reduce food allergies dramatically. In fact, there is little evidence that lectins, other than a handful of exceptions, present a problem for most people.

To conclude our discussion of lectins, let me offer some perspective. If the argument is that because "some" lectins are toxic to "some" people, then "all" people should avoid "all" lectins, we have a problem. We live in a world where food exists as part of a chain, with predators eating prey – and the prey develops defenses to protect itself from being eaten. Lectins are part of the circle of life and can't be avoided; they permeate the food chain as predator eats prey. This means that if you wish to avoid all lectins, you would have to avoid all food, since all food contains lectins. To do otherwise implies selective belief in your theory.

So, what should we eat on the Paleo Diet?

Meat (particularly organ meats such as liver and kidneys), poultry, and fish top the list. Remember, we're talking about "hunter" gatherers. In fact, according to some proponents, flesh should provide upwards of 65% of the calories in a Paleo Diet, with fruits and vegetables providing only about 35%. Eggs are also big on the diet.

Fruits and vegetables

Fruit and root vegetables such as carrots, turnips, and beets are okay, but not tubers such as potatoes, sweet potatoes, and yams. Incidentally, I find the exclusion of tubers requires a bit of theoretical bending. The argument is that potatoes are a "new world" crop and humans have only been eating them for maybe the last 35,000 years. But in truth, yams are an African crop that people have been eating since the dawn of time. So why are they excluded? And if that's your logic for excluding potatoes, then why is turkey okay? After all, turkey is a "new world" species, not even introduced into Europe until the 16th Century.

As for fruits, berries of all kinds are good — strawberries, blueberries, and raspberries etc. are good. From there, differences in Paleo's abound. Tree fruits are controversial. For example, some say apples are great. Others call them "bags of sugar." And still others say they're okay if you eat the low sugar varieties. And yet, if the theory is based on eating what hunter-gathers ate, then tree fruits would have to be top of the charts. Not to go Biblical, but I think it's pretty safe to say that tree fruits such as apples and pomegranates have been part of the human diet since the very first man and woman walked the earth. And I don't believe hunter gatherers selected their fruit based on the glycemic index.

Also, fruits contain lectins — just like grains. Apricots, bananas, cherries, kiwis, melons, papayas, peaches, pineapples, plums, and even berries are all known to contain lectins and cause allergies. In fact, fruit allergies make up about 10 percent of all food related allergies. So why are fruits allowed? Incidentally, new research has shown that allergies to fruit are actually made possible by pectin, the soluble fiber found in fruit. The pectin surrounds the fruit allergens in the digestive tract so that they don't get broken down and enter the bloodstream intact. Using a digestive enzyme supplement that contains added pectinase can help moderate that problem by breaking down the fruit pectin, which then exposes the allergens to digestive juices and enzymes.

Nuts and legumes

Curiously, nuts are cool on the diet — pretty much all nuts except cashews and peanuts, which are actually beans. Yes, I understand that people have eaten gathered nuts since the beginning of the human race, but if allergenic lectins are your thing, nuts should be a "no no." Tree nuts including macadamia nuts, brazil nuts, almonds, walnuts, pecans, pistachios, chestnuts, hazelnuts, and pine nuts are high in allergenic lectins. And unlike grain allergies, which tend to be low level and chronic, tree nut allergies tend to be severe, and are strongly associated with anaphylaxis and even death. Walnuts (and cashews) top the list for the tree nuts most likely to cause an allergic reaction. Peanuts, incidentally, are legumes, which is why they are on the Paleo no-no list. As legumes, they are biologically unrelated to tree nuts; nevertheless, there is a high level of cross-allergenic reactivity between peanuts and tree nuts. So again, if peanuts are not allowed, why are tree nuts okay? I'm just looking for consistency in the theory behind the Paleo Diet and its application in the real world.

Another factor to consider is that tree nuts have the same enzyme blockers that seeds and grains have, and for the same reason — to prevent premature sprouting. And like seeds, grains, and legumes, those enzymes are neutralized by soaking in water and exposure to heat. But that goes against the premise behind the Paleo Diet. So once again, we have to ask, "Why nuts?"

Incidentally, sprouting nuts will eliminate most of the blocking enzymes as well as many of the allergenic lectins.

Legumes, or beans, present much the same problem. They have blocking enzymes to prevent premature sprouting and toxins to keep predators away. Soaking and cooking will pretty much eliminate that problem, but because they have to be cooked, they violate the "Paleolithic theory" of no cooking and so are not allowed.

Are you kidding me?

I find the theory behind the Paleo Diet to be somewhat distorting of facts and highly inconsistent within its own logic. We've discussed a number of those inconsistencies already and will explore several more in a moment. However, it is important to keep in mind that **just because an underlying theory may be wrong does not mean that the program itself is without value**. So once again, let me state that theory aside, the Paleo Diet has much to recommend it. But before we go there, let's examine a few more of the theoretical inconsistencies.

Location, location, location

The assumed diet of the hunter-gatherers modeled by the Paleo's is reflective of cave people living in Northern Europe in cold climes where plants did not readily grow. But the simple truth is that hunter-gatherer societies in other locations ate decidedly different diets. As Katharine

Milton points out in an editorial in the *American Journal of Clinical Nutrition*:

"The Kung might live in conditions close to the "ideal" hunting and gathering environment. What do the Kung eat? Animal foods are estimated to contribute 33% and plant foods 67% of their daily energy intakes. Fifty percent (by wt.) of their plant-based diet comes from the mongongo nut, which is available throughout the year in massive quantities. Similarly, the hunter-gatherer Hadza of Tanzania consume "the bulk of their diet" as wild plants, although they live in an area with an exceptional abundance of game animals and refer to themselves as hunters."4

And it's not just modern examples of hunter-gatherer tribes. There is solid evidence that suggests that Paleolithic peoples commonly ate grain, and even flour, as far back as 30,000 years ago._In fact, there is quite reasonable evidence that people were processing cereal grains for food as much as 200,000 years ago. The bottom line is that the fundamental premise that Paleolithic peoples did not eat grains and that they ate large amounts of meat is only "suggested" by historical records, not necessarily supported by them.

Another example is salt. Salt is a taboo in most Paleo Diets, and yet the evidence is that the people of the Lenggong Valley in Malaysia were not only eating salt 200,000 years ago, but had created tools for grinding it. And animals will eat/lick salt whenever they find it. Virtually all animals consume it. Salt is actually an interesting test for the Paleo Diet. Animals eat it. Cavemen ate it. And yet, it's taboo in the Paleo Diet. Obviously, the Paleo Dieters' faith in their ancestors' food choices only goes so far.

On May 4th 2011, the *Journal of the American Medical Association* published these results of a study done on people and salt. **Stunningly, the study found that participants with the lowest salt intake had the highest rate of death from heart disease during the follow up (4 percent), and people who ate the most salt had the lowest (less than 1 percent).** In the case of salt, cavemen really did know better; unfortunately, advocates of the Paleo diet, despite their professed belief in the caveman diet, backed the wrong horse: bad science.

Anatomical imperative

Another problem I have is that just because people ate certain foods does not necessarily mean that those were the best foods to eat — merely that those were most likely the foods that were easiest to obtain in their local environment. If you were living in Europe on the edge of a glacier, mangoes were not part of your diet, not because they were unhealthy, but because they were not readily available. On the other hand, if you grew up in the Indus valley 100,000 years ago, a vegetarian diet would have been a strong option because fruits and vegetables would have been readily available.

As anyone who has been to college knows, you don't live on pizza and beer while attending school because they are a "natural" part of your diet; you live on them because they are readily available on campus and all your friends are eating them.

To me, a much better indicator of what foods we are designed to eat is your digestive tract. Animals that eat particular foods have digestive tracts designed to handle those foods. Carnivores have sharp teeth for ripping and tearing flesh, and short digestive tracts for quickly eliminating waste once digested in the stomach — so it doesn't have time to putrefy in the intestines. (Meat putrefies.) Animals that eat plants have flat teeth for grinding and long digestive systems to allow time to extract nutrients from plant matter, which does not putrefy. Human digestive systems largely match Chimpanzees, who eat mostly fruits and nuts and termites, but will eat a small amount of monkey meat when they can get it.

Premise of health is arbitrary

The idea that the so-called Paleo Diet is inherently healthier is simply not supported by the evidence, either ancient or modern. What is supported is that eating modern highly processed, high-glycemic foods is unhealthy. Diabetes was virtually unknown in China until people began eating the modern Western diet. But before people started eating modern diets in China, they weren't eating anything remotely close to the Paleo Diet. They were eating a largely vegetarian diet grounded in rice and noodles.

For centuries, they ate grains without problems. It was the introduction of refined sugars and oils and processed fast foods "what did them in," to quote Eliza Doolittle. As a side note, although meat consumption has gone up dramatically in China, with disease rates climbing right alongside them, it's probably not the meat that's causing the problem. It's most likely all of the refined, processed, fast food that's killing them. Then again, one of the most comprehensive diet studies ever conducted, known as the China Study, touched on this issue in some detail — coming down in favor of the vegetarian diet.

When T. Colin Campbell's *The China Study* was released in 2006, it quickly rocketed to best seller status primarily propelled by word of mouth given its small, relatively unknown publisher not exactly renowned for works of scientific rigor.

In short order, *The China Study* became firmly established as the de facto nutritional bible of the plant based diet posse. A similar phenomenon has occurred with the 2017 release of the Netflix documentary *What The Health.*

At first blush, *The China Study* seems so utterly credible – so bulletproof if you will.

Unfortunately, like much of the nutritional dogma presented today all in the name of supposedly scientific rigor, *The China Study* is actually far from it with misrepresented data the order of the day.

Perhaps the biggest hole in Campbell's work is one that he identified himself in one of his own scientific papers published only two years before *The China Study.* Despite Campbell's claim that near vegan rural Chinese exhibit superior health to those consuming animal foods, the paper concludes from the epidemiological survey of 6500 subjects from 65 rural counties in China:

"it is the largely vegetarian, inland communities who have the greatest all risk mortalities and morbidities and who have the lowest LDL cholesterols."

Whoops! Campbell finds that "... the protective effect of fish consumption as validated by red cell DHA is universal." It doesn't look like that large epidemiological analysis known as The China Study is so compelling regarding the benefits of plant-based diets after all!

Now, a new study involving over one hundred thousand subjects further bolsters the argument that animal proteins are not the ticking time bomb to your health so erroneously argued by Campbell.

Meat Eating Inversely Associated with Death from Cancer and Heart Disease

The *American Journal of Clinical Nutrition* published in July 2013 the results of a huge analysis of ecological data from the United Nations comparing country-specific meat consumption in Asia, specifically the countries of Bangladesh, China, Japan, Korea, and Taiwan.

112,310 men and 184,411 women were followed for 6.6 to 15.6 years. During that time, 24,283 all-cause, 9558 cancer, and 6373 cardiovascular disease (CVD) deaths were recorded.

The researchers concluded that while meat intake in Asian countries has increased in recent years, there was no evidence of a higher risk of mortality as a result. In fact, the analysis provided evidence of an inverse association with red meat, poultry, and fish/seafood consumption and cardiovascular mortality in men and cancer mortality in women!

This means that higher meat consumption has actually been correlated with fewer heart disease deaths in Asian men and fewer cancer deaths in Asian women:

"Red meat intake was inversely associated with CVD mortality in men and with cancer mortality in women in Asian countries."

It seems the vegan bible has suffered yet another blow to its cherry-picked conclusions. Unlike *The China "Study"*, this large analysis of Asian ecological data is a Real Study published in a Real (peer-reviewed) Scientific Journal. Not a blockbuster work of fiction designed to sell books through promotion of outrageous black and white nutritional propaganda.

What meat are we talking about?

The meat promoted in the Paleo Diet is not necessarily the same as the meat that was available way back when. While it is true that some Paleo advocates advise eating only lean cuts of meat that are either hunted in the wild, or grass-fed, most do not. And in fact, most people following the diet opt for lean cuts bought in regular grocery stores — primarily because of convenience and cost. But grocery store meat, pork, and poultry come with a wide range of "bonus" goodies not found in Paleolithic times, including:

- Growth hormones
- Antibiotics
- High pesticide concentrations
- Heavy metals
- Toxicity from over 100,000 manmade chemicals now found in the environment
- High levels of omega-6 fatty acids as a result of being grain fattened
- Not to mention the fact that cancerous and tumorous meat is not necessarily removed at the slaughterhouse, and may quite easily find its way to the butcher's shop. If you think the USDA is actively preventing sick animals from entering the food supply, think again. Unbelievable abuses have been documented happening under the very noses of USDA inspectors.

As for fish, even if you catch it yourself, you're now looking at mercury contamination, dioxin, and sex altering hormones — things Paleo fishermen never had to deal with.

Germs in meat

And now there's something else to watch for in today's meat. Scientists from Arizona's Translational Genomics Research Institute recently announced that 47 percent of samples of beef, pork, and poultry obtained from supermarkets around the country tested positive for Staphylococcus aureus, the bacteria that causes staph infections — and 52% of those bugs were resistant to at least three kinds of antibiotics. S. Aureus already kills about 11,000 people in the U.S. every year. Thanks to contaminated meat, we can look for that number to climb.9

Cooking meat

Most Paleo's cook their meat, even though cooking is the knock against grains — one of those inconsistencies we try not to think too much about. Nevertheless, there is a small subset of Paleo's who believe that humans have not adapted to cooked foods, even though the evidence is that cavemen were cooking their meat almost since day one. And so, this subset of Paleo's eats only foods which are both raw and early Paleolithic. Actresses such as Uma Thurman, Demi Moore, and Natalie Portman are/were believers. The concept is not without science. Cooking meat creates heterocyclic amines (HCAs), which have been linked to cancer. The higher the temperature used in cooking and the more the meat is cooked, the greater the risk. One study out of the National Cancer Institute's Division of Cancer Epidemiology and Genetics found that people who eat their beef medium-well or well-done have more than a 300% greater risk of stomach cancer than those who eat their beef rare or medium-rare. And yet another study linked the consumption of well-done meat to higher rates of breast cancer. But there's good news for diehard carnivores who love a cook-out or a tailgate party. More recent studies have confirmed that marinating meat sharply reduces the level of HCAs when you are cooking — making it much safer. I'll bet that's something cavemen didn't know.

In any case, the evidence for when man first started cooking with fire ranges from 230,000 years ago (confirmed) to evidence at archeological sites in Spain and France that strongly indicate dates ranging from 300,000 to as many as 500,000 years ago — with cooked rhinoceroses' meat on the menu.

All in all, this brings up three conundrums.

- Since most cave people cooked their meat, eating raw meat denies the foundation of the Paleo Diet — i.e., eating what cavemen ate.
- On the other hand, if you do cook your meat, then you're doing something potentially unhealthy, which denies the premise of the Paleo Diet — that if cavemen did it, it's good for you.
- And when did people first start marinating meat, which makes cooked meat healthier — something that certainly started happening after the Paleolithic era?

Evaluation

So, after all is said and done, where do I stand on the Paleo Diet?

As I said at the outset, there is much to recommend it. I'm all for cutting back on sugar and dairy. And as for grains, I'm all for cutting way back on those too. Considering the negatives associated with the excessive consumption of grains (most notably associated with high glycemic responses and allergies), On the other hand, consumption of certain grains in moderation, if selected carefully, can provide significant health benefits with little downside. For example, sprouted grains and cereal grasses have all the positives associated with grains and virtually none of the negatives. Think wheatgrass juice. And let's quickly single out barley, maybe the king of grains. It's high in beta-glucans; it's one of the least acidic grains; and it's one of the lowest of all foods on the glycemic index. And when consumed in its sprouted, pre-sprouted, or cereal grass forms, it's a monster of nutrition.

I also have a fundamental problem with the consumption of high levels of meat. All meats, fish, poultry, and eggs are acid forming in the body. When metabolized, the proteins produce sulfuric acid and phosphoric acid. And fats produce acetic acid. The way the body handles them is to neutralize them by converting them into acid salts by combining them with the minerals sodium, calcium, potassium, and magnesium. Of these, calcium is the most important.

Now, here's the key: your body uses a priority system if there are not enough available minerals to neutralize all of the acids present. After extracting what it can from urine and soft tissues (creating a rich environment for the spread of cancer), your body turns to its great mineral bank — your bones. So, if your diet is too acid-forming, your body will fairly quickly begin to leach calcium from your bones to balance the low pH and avoid death. In effect, your body says osteoporosis is preferable to death.

And in fact, osteoporosis is seen to start earlier in "pre-contact" Inuit, who relied heavily on whale and seal meat, then in the Eskimos eating a more modern diet, "post-contact."13 Even better, Masai warriors in Africa also partake of a high meat diet and begin developing osteoporosis in their 20's. The women of the tribe do not share in the high meat diet, and do not show early signs of osteoporosis. But keep in mind, meat is by no means the sole determinant of osteoporosis, and in fact its negative effects can be easily mitigated by higher consumption of offsetting minerals such as calcium, potassium, and magnesium, and through the use of weight bearing exercise to strengthen the bones. But high meat consumption is a contributing factor.

And one last issue concerns intestinal flora. High levels of meat in the diet disrupt the balance of beneficial bacteria in the intestinal tract. First, virtually all meat, chicken, and pork that you eat (other than organic) is loaded with antibiotics, which destroy all of the beneficial bacteria in your gastrointestinal tract. But that aside, heavy consumption of meat (of any purity) significantly compromises beneficial bacteria in the colon, resulting in a 1,000 percent increase in the levels of harmful bacteria and a 90 percent drop in the levels of beneficial bacteria.

In addition, epidemiological studies done at Harvard Medical School show that, "Men who eat red meat as a main dish five or more times a week have four times the risk of colon cancer than men who eat red meat less than once a month." They are also more than twice as likely to get prostate cancer. And a recent study found that women who had more than one-and-a-half servings of red meat a day doubled their risk of hormone receptor—positive breast cancer.14 To be sure, studies such as these do not differentiate between the consumption of hormone-laced commercial beef and organic grass-fed beef, which might produce decidedly different results. But a cautionary flag has certainly been raised.

Recommendations

As I said, just because the theory behind the diet may be questionable, does not mean that there is not much to take from the diet. I absolutely agree with the following:

- Cut way back or eliminate all grains. And if you eat grains, opt for hypoallergenic grains that have been soaked, sprouted, or well cooked.
- Eliminate all high omega-6 store bought oils from your diet. For low temperature cooking, use olive oil and coconut oil. For high

temperature cooking, use avocado oil, grape seed oil, or rice bran oil. Supplement with omega-3 fatty acids.

- Eliminate all added sugars.
- When eating fruit, lean more towards berries than tree fruit; they're higher in antioxidants. But there's no need to be afraid of eating tree fruit, which tends to be higher in soluble fiber.
- Cut back or eliminate all beans, and if you eat them, make sure you soak them before cooking, and then cook them well before eating.
- Nuts are fine if you're not allergic. Use whole fresh nuts that have been soaked/sprouted. Do not use pasteurized or "roasted" nuts — especially those roasted in oil.
- Cut way back on white potatoes, but yams and sweet potatoes are okay in moderation.
- Eliminate all commercial dairy from your diet. And if you do opt for some dairy, choose raw dairy despite what the government says — or at the very least opt for organic, grass-fed dairy.
- If you eat meat, use only organic, grass-fed meat. And keep consumption to less than 4 oz a day. And don't overcook it. (And here you're faced with another conundrum if you eat commercial meat. If you undercook it, you face the risk of bacterial infection. If you overcook it, you face the risk of cancer. If you want to eat medium rare meat, you're going to have to buy organic, grass-fed meat from a supplier you trust.)

As I said before, the Paleo Diet has much to recommend it. But then again, isn't what I've described above really just a very clean Mediterranean Diet — light on grains, meat and dairy — heavy on fresh vegetables, clean fish, and fruit.

Sounds good to me.

Why Antibiotics and Antivirals Fail

In one of the latest issues of the CDC's Morbidity and Mortality Weekly Report features a story about a deadly bacterial illness commonly seen in people on antibiotics but that now appears to be growing more common in patients not taking such drugs. The bacterium is Clostridium difficile (d fee seal), also known as C-diff. Its symptoms include diarrhea, fever, abdominal pain, loss of appetite and nausea, and last year it was blamed for 100 deaths over 18 months in just one hospital in Quebec, Canada. And in a second article in the New England Journal of Medicine, health officials said samples of the same bacteria taken from eight US hospitals show it's mutating to become even more resistant to antibiotics. Especially disturbing, according to the Centers for Disease Control and Prevention, recent cases in four states indicate it's now appearing more often in healthy people who have not been admitted to health-care facilities or even taken antibiotics. The bottom line is that C-diff has grown resistant to antibiotics that work against other colon bacteria. How did this happen? Quite simply, when patients took those antibiotics, particularly clindamycin, competing bacteria died off and C-diff exploded.

But this chapter isn't about C-diff. C-diff is merely the headline trigger. What I want to talk about is why and how bacteria like C-diff and viruses like bird flu develop resistance to antibiotics and antiviral drugs. And more importantly...what you can do about it.

Antibiotic Resistant Infections

Penicillin was discovered (actually rediscovered) by Dr. Alexander Fleming in 1928. But just four years after drug companies began mass-producing it in 1943, microbes began appearing that could resist it. Since then, we've seen penicillin-resistant strains of pneumonia, gonorrhea, and hospital-acquired intestinal infections join the list. And it's not just penicillin. Bacteria resistant to most of the other antibiotics of choice have also appeared and proliferated on a regular basis.

Antibiotic resistance to man-made drugs is almost impossible to stop since it is the result of some simple rules of evolution. Any population of organisms, bacteria included, naturally includes variants with unusual traits — in this case, the ability to withstand a particular antibiotic's attack. When said antibiotic is used and kills the defenseless bacteria, it leaves behind those bacteria that can resist it. These renegade variants then multiply, increasing their numbers a million-fold in a single day, instantly becoming the dominant variant. In other words, the very act of using an antibiotic creates the opportunity for strains resistant to it to flourish.

How do antibiotics work?

It's important to understand that antibiotics vary in the way they kill microbes. Penicillin, for example, kills bacteria by attaching to their cell walls and then breeching those walls, thus killing the bacteria. Erythromycin, tetracycline, and streptomycin, on the other hand, kill bacteria by attacking the structures inside the bacteria (ribosomes) that allow them to make proteins, thus also destroying the bacteria.

Unfortunately, because each antibiotic is a single compound and one dimensional in its approach, it's not that hard for microbes to "evolve" around such attacks. For example, microbes resistant to penicillin have developed cell walls different from the norm and that prevent the penicillin from binding. Similarly, other variants prevent antibiotics from binding to ribosomes, thus neutralize the effect of those antibiotics.

Again, because antibiotics are one dimensional in their approach, it's not that hard for microbes to "evolve" around them.

Where it gets really frightening, though, is that bacteria swap genes like politician's swap favors — which brings us to vancomycin, the antibiotic of last resort. When all other antibiotics failed, doctors knew they could count on vancomycin. But then vancomycin resistance was discovered in a common hospital microbe, enterococcus. By 1991, 38 hospitals in the United States reported the variant. Just one year later, vancomycin resistant Staph bacteria were observed with the same gene. What this means is that not only are bacteria programmed to "evolve" defenses against antibiotics, but once they produce such a defense, they are also programmed to rapidly share that defense with other bacteria — thus rapidly spreading the resistance.

Viruses

Whereas bacteria are single-celled organisms, viruses are far simpler — more primitive even. Essentially, viruses consist of one type of biochemical (a nucleic acid, such as DNA or RNA) wrapped in another (protein). Viruses are so primitive, in fact, that most biologists do not consider them to be living things, but instead, they are considered infectious particles. Since antibiotics specifically attack bacteria, they are useless against viruses. For viruses, doctors rely on a much less effective group of drugs called antivirals. Tamiflu, which governments are currently stockpiling as bird flu insurance, is one such antiviral.

Because of their primitive structure, viruses mutate even more easily than bacteria. Whereas antibiotics can remain effective for 2-5 years before resistant strains render them ineffective, antiviral resistant strains can appear in a matter of months, or even weeks. And in fact, we have seen that with Tamiflu. Although governments are stockpiling it as a safety net for bird flu, bird flu arrived on the scene pretty much resistant to Tamiflu and the other antivirals right out of the gate. And even those flu's that Tamiflu was once helpful with are developing resistant strains by the month.

What can science do?

It was briefly thought that alternating the most commonly used antibiotics might stop the spread of antibiotic resistance. But a new model shows that the practice of cycling, alternating between two or more classes of antibiotics as often as every few months, probably will not work.

The latest theory is that mixing cocktails of antibiotics may help. And, in fact, this is closer to the way natural substances avoid the resistance problem.

How natural substances avoid the problem

When you think about how quickly pathogens "evolve around" antibiotic and antiviral drugs, it's more than amazing that they have been unable to do so against most natural anti-pathogens such as garlic, olive leaf, and oil of oregano even given tens of thousands of years to do so. How does this happen? What is their secret?

Actually, it's quite simple – or more accurately, quite complex. Earlier, I spoke about how drugs are essentially one dimensional, which allows microbes an easy avenue to evolve around them. Natural anti-pathogens, on the other hand, are anything but one dimensional. They often contain dozens of bio-chemicals. Not all of them are "active," of course, but many of the so called non-active bio-chemicals work to potentiate the active ones and offer combinations with each other numbering in the thousands – presenting a complexity that makes it virtually impossible for microbes to work around.

Take garlic for example

For a long time, many people thought there was only one active component in garlic, allicin (in fact, many companies still promote that concept). It was believed that raw garlic had very little biological activity, but when you "damage" garlic cloves - by slicing, cooking, or chewing them - the enzyme alliinase immediately converts non-active alliin into the active ingredient, allicin.

As I mentioned, it was once thought that allicin was garlic's principal active ingredient. However, researchers now know that allicin is rapidly oxidized. In the process of oxidation, allicin breaks down into more than 100 biologically active sulfur-containing compounds. While allicin may still serve as a general marker of garlic's potency, research increasingly points to S-allylcysteine (ally syst a hene) and other compounds as the most therapeutically active ingredients in garlic.

So how many possible pathogenic defense combinations can you get from garlic's 100 biologically active compounds? A whole bunch!! Thousands and thousands and thousands, in fact!

With 100 objects/compounds to work with and possible combinations ranging from any 2 of them to any 99 of them, the complexity is just far, far, far too much for simple pathogens to evolve around.

And that's the secret. But it gets even better.

When you combine several natural substances in one formula, the combinations of compounds are beyond counting. Quite simply, microbes cannot evolve around them. Let's look at a few.

Onion

Everything that's been said about Garlic can be said about onion. Onions and garlic share many of the same powerful sulfur bearing compounds that work so effectively as anti-viral and anti-bacterial agents.

Ginger

Ginger has been traditionally used to treat colds and flu. Chinese studies have shown that ginger helps kill influenza viruses (even avian flu), and an Indian report shows that it increases the immune system's ability to fight infection.

Olive Leaf Extract

Olive leaf extract has a long history of being used against illnesses in which microorganisms play a major role. In more recent years, a drug company discovered that in vitro (in a test tube), an extract from olive leaf (calcium elenolate) was effective in eliminating a very broad range of organisms, including bacteria, viruses, parasites, and yeast/mold/fungus. https://www.npscript.com/dougcaporrino/olive-leaf-capsules/GA0093PAR#undefined2

Habañero and Horseradish

These are stimulants that quicken and excite the body. They energize the body (helping it to marshal its defenses against invading viruses). In addition, they help to carry blood to all parts of the body.

They are also diaphoretics and thus help raise the temperature of the body, which increases the activity of the body's immune system.

Horseradish, in particular, contains volatile oils that are similar to those found in mustard. In test tubes, the volatile oils in horseradish have shown antibiotic properties, which may account for its effectiveness in treating throat and upper respiratory tract infections. At levels attainable in human urine after taking the volatile oil of horseradish, the oil has been shown to kill bacteria that can cause urinary tract infections, and one early trial found that horseradish extract may be a useful treatment for people with urinary tract infections.

Liquid Ionic Zinc

Like colloidal silver, liquid zinc is both anti-bacterial and anti-viral, but without the potential toxicity issues found with silver. Zinc is found in all body fluids, including the moisture in the eyes, lungs, nose, urine, and saliva. Proper zinc levels offer a defense against the entrance of pathogens. In the 1800's, surgeons used zinc as an antiseptic/antibiotic after surgery; they noted it's amazing healing properties. Wounds would heal, at times, as quickly as 24 hours after an operation, without swelling, and scarring was barely noticeable after a short period of time. https://www.npscript.com/dougcaporrino/liquid-ionic-zinc-50mg/TR0025PAR

Oil of Wild Mountain Oregano

Numerous studies have shown wild mountain oregano oil (not to be confused with the oregano found in your kitchen) to be a potent antimicrobial. It has been proven useful as an antiviral, antibacterial, and antifungal agent rivaling even pharmaceutical antibiotics such as streptomycin, penicillin, vacnomycin, and nystatin, in its ability to eliminate microbes. Remarkably it accomplishes this without promoting the development of drug resistant strains and other problems often attributed to the use of standard antibiotics. In addition to this already impressive list of abilities Oregano Oil is also a powerful parasitic expellant. https://www.npscript.com/dougcaporrino/oil-of-oregano-capsules/GA0094PAR

Grapefruit Seed Extract

Grapefruit seed extract was originally developed as an antiparasitic, but studies quickly showed that it had the ability to inhibit the growth of not only parasites, but fungi, viruses, and bacteria as well. The active ingredients of grapefruit seed extract are non-toxic and are synthesized from the seed and pulp of certified organically grown grapefruit. The process converts the grapefruit bioflavonoids (polyphenolics) into an extremely potent compound that is being used to kill strep, staph, salmonella, E. Coli, candida, herpes, influenza, parasites, fungi, and more. https://www.npscript.com/dougcaporrino/grapefruit-seed-extract-400mg/DN0293PAR

Apple-Cider Vinegar

ACV (Apple-Cider Vinegar) serves several functions:

- It's the tincture medium for the formula, as opposed to alcohol (which is the tincture medium in an immune tonic).
- ACV is anathema to all kinds of germs that attack the throat. In effect, it acts like a sponge and draws out throat germs and toxins from the surrounding tissue.
- And finally, ACV stimulates a condition called antipathogen (Asa tall issis) in which toxic wastes that are harmful to the body are broken down and rendered harmless.

https://bragg.com/products/bragg-organic-apple-cider-vinegar.html

Conclusion

As I said, individually, the effectiveness of these ingredients is astonishing. But taken as a whole, and when you consider the number of possible active biochemical combinations these 10 ingredients and their hundreds of biochemical compounds afford, it would take bacteria and viruses more time than the earth has left in existence to evolve their way around them.

DMSO - The Real Miracle Solution

In 1866, Russian scientist Alexander Saytzeff isolated a most curious and peculiar chemical compound. It was crystalline, odor-less, non-toxic and had a garlic-like taste when consumed. At the time, he had no way to predict that his discovery was going to prove highly controversial throughout its entire medical history, that it was going to be tested in thousands of studies and provide miraculous relief for numerous patients.

I'm talking here about *dimethyl sulfoxide* (DMSO), an organic sulfur compound which was used only as an industrial solvent, that is, until its medical properties were discovered in 1963 by a research team headed by Stanley W. Jacob, MD.

DMSO is a by-product of Kraft pulping (the 'sulfate process') which converts wood into wood pulp leaving almost pure cellulose fibers. As industrial as it may sound, the process simply entails a treatment of wood chips with a mixture of sodium hydroxide and sodium sulfide, known as white liquor, breaking the bonds which link lignin (from the Latin word lignum, meaning wood) to the cellulose.

DMSO is useful as a pain reliever and also in burns, acne, arthritis, mental retardation, strokes, head injury, scleroderma, it soothes toothaches, eases headaches, hemorrhoids, muscle strains, it prevents paralysis from spinal-cord injuries and softens scar tissues. In fact, it is useful in well over 300 ailments and is safe to use. You might think that a compound that has so many alleged uses and benefits should be automatically suspect, so let's have a close look at its properties and the data available and we'll shed some light in this miraculous chemical.

Sulfur: The Stuff of Life

DMSO is an intermediate product of the global Sulfur Cycle which distributes bioavailable sulfur for all animal and plant life (Parcell, 2002). Sulfur compounds are found in all body cells and are indispensable for life, they are needed for a number of chemical reactions involved in the detoxification of drugs and other harmful toxins, and they have potential clinical applications in the treatment of a number of conditions such as depression, fibromyalgia, arthritis, interstitial cystitis, athletic injuries, congestive heart failure, diabetes, cancer, and AIDS (Parcell, 2002). Among the sulfur compounds, DMSO is probably the one that has the widest range and greatest number of therapeutic applications ever shown for any other single chemical. It has around 40 pharmacological properties that may be beneficial in the prevention, relief or reversal of numerous diseases (Morton, 1993).

Someone complained to Dr. Jacob of a splitting headache and gave him permission to apply some DMSO after hearing of its capabilities. The headache was gone in minutes, came back in four hours, and left for good after DMSO was applied a second time. Used for one purpose, sometimes it did another; put on a cold sore, within a few hours it cleared up a woman's sinusitis. A woman who had had a stroke found after DMSO was painted on her painful jaw that she could now write with her paralyzed hand and could walk better. (Haley, 2000)

Therapeutic Properties

DMSO is an effective pain killer, blocking nerve conduction fibers that produce pain. It reduces inflammation and swelling by reducing inflammatory chemicals. It improves blood supply to an area of injury by dilating blood vessels and increasing delivery of oxygen and by reducing blood platelet stickiness. It stimulates healing, which is a key to its usefulness in any condition. It is among the most potent free radical scavengers known to man, if not the most potent one. This is a crucial mechanism since some molecules in our bodies produce an unequal number of electrons and the instability of the number causes them to destroy other cells. DMSO hooks on to those molecules and they are then expelled from the body with the DMSO.

DR. Stanley Jacob working with DMSO in the 1960s

DMSO also penetrates the skin and the blood-brain barrier with ease, penetrating tissues, and entering the bloodstream. Furthermore, DMSO protects the cells from mechanical damage and less of it is needed to achieve results as time passes as opposed to most pharmaceuticals where increasing doses are required. It has a calming effect in the central nervous system and it reaches all areas of the body, when absorbed through the skin, including the brain. That is, DMSO applied to one area often leads to pain relief in some other location due to its systemic effect.

It acts as a carrier for other substances or drugs and it also potentiates their effect. In fact, certain drugs dissolved in DMSO, such as antibiotics and insulin, may be used in a lower dose than usual without reducing their therapeutic efficacy and in addition, their undesirable side effects are greatly diminished. Also, drugs are able to pass through the blood-brain barrier which is usually impenetrable.

DMSO promotes the excretion of urine and functions as a muscle relaxant. It boosts the immune system, increasing the production of white cells and macrophages that destroy foreign material and pathogens in the body. It also has anti-bacterial, anti-viral and anti-fungal properties. DMSO also increases the permeability of cell membranes, allowing a flushing of toxins from the cell.

As a source of sulfur, DMSO aids in heavy metal detoxification. Sulfur binds with toxic heavy metals (mercury, lead, aluminum, cadmium, arsenic, nickel) and eliminates them via urination, defecation and sweating.

FDA and Big Pharma Obstacles

DMSO is sold in health food stores, mail-order outlets, on the Internet, and in most countries around the world. It is used by millions for its health benefits yet in the U.S., DMSO has FDA approval only as a preservative of stem cells, bone marrow cells, and organs for transplant, and for interstitial cystitis - a painful inflammatory condition of the bladder which is very difficult to treat with other therapies.

That DMSO has not found favor as a remedy for other medical conditions is partly due to the inability to test it in double-blind experiments. Blind studies, as the name suggests, requires that a study be done without knowing which patient is taking the placebo or the drug. In the case of the DMSO, a blind study is impossible since the peculiar garlic-like taste and smell (no matter the route of application) gives it away and no satisfactory placebo could be devised that would mimic this particular effect of DMSO (Steinberg, 1967).

The FDA and 'big pharma' would prefer we remain dependent on their drugs

If you search for DMSO on the U.S. National Library of Medicine (pubmed.gov), you'll get almost 30,000 indexed results, making it one of the most studied compounds of our time. Yet, we are led to believe that DMSO can't pass the required regulations for its approval in other medical conditions even though its effectiveness and low toxicity profile is unquestionable.

You see, DMSO is a common chemical that can be manufactured cheaply. No drug company can get an exclusive patent since it is also a natural compound, therefore there is no significant financial return. In fact, an executive of a major drug company is quoted as saying, "I don't care if DMSO is the major drug of our century **and we all know it is**, it isn't worth it to us" [CBS TV show 60 minutes with Mike Wallace, The Riddle of DMSO]. If DMSO were to be approved by the FDA, it would be competitive and drug companies would be unable to hold the patents. In the words of the director of the Bureau of Drugs of the FDA, J. Richard

Crout, M.D., "DMSO is a low toxicity and safe compound (...) I think that it is a fact of life that drug companies are not going to invest in something unless they think there is some financial return" [CBS TV show *60 minutes* with Mike Wallace, *The Riddle of DMSO*].

Despite restrictions on the use of DMSO, thousands of Americans purchase it on the 'black market' each year, its popularity due not to publicity, but rather 'word of mouth'. When you have something that relieves all kinds of ailments, including some life-threatening ones, people naturally recommend it to friends and family!

Quick Guide and Ailments

DMSO is generally applied to the skin in a gel, cream, or liquid. It can be taken by mouth or as an intravenous injection, in many cases along with other drugs. It has also been administered subcutaneously, intramuscularly, and, by inhalation, instilled into the eye, on the mucous membranes, and into the urinary bladder. Strengths and dosages vary widely.

DMSO being distilled

If you are just dealing with pain or an injury, use a topical application. Don't drink it. Drinking it is for serious detoxing and other internal necessities. If you use a rose scented DMSO cream, chances are that nobody will be able to smell DMSO's garlic-like smell.

The usual oral dose of DMSO is one teaspoon per day of DMSO 70% (Morton, 1993). But since it can trigger detoxification reactions and DMSO's total excretion from the body can take several days, it is best to do it only once a week. Start with half a teaspoon of DMSO 50% and increase to a teaspoon of DMSO 70% only if any possible detoxification reaction is well tolerated.

When you use liquid DMSO in the skin, let it dry for over 20 to 30 minutes before wiping the rest out. The skin must be clean, dry, and unbroken for any topical use of DMSO. The face and the neck are more sensitive to DMSO and no higher concentrations than 50% should be applied there. Topical concentrations of DMSO should be kept below

70% in areas where there is a reduction of circulation. When 60 to 90% DMSO is applied to the skin, warmth, redness, itching, and sometimes local hives may occur. This usually disappears within a couple of hours and using natural aloe vera, gel or cream, will help counteract or prevent this effect. When 60 to 90% DMSO is applied to the palm on the hand, the skin may wrinkle and stay that way for several days.

Common health problems for which people will apply topical DMSO at home include acute musculoskeletal injuries and inflammations. The earlier DMSO is used, the more dramatic the result. A 70% concentration of DMSO mixed with water in volumes ranging from 8 to 12 ml, applied on and around the injury in a wide area at least three times daily, will have a healing affect in 4 out of 5 people.

Arthritis, Sprains, Strains

It provides rapid relief of pain and increased mobility and reduction of inflammation when used topically. You can see a positive response within 5 to 20 minutes and usually lasting for 4 to 6 hours. (Steinberg, 1967).

the calcification disappeared. (Haley, 2000)

Stroke

Given soon after a stroke, DMSO can dissolve the clot that causes the stroke, restoring circulation and avoiding paralysis. Once DMSO gets into the body either daubed on the skin, given in I.V., or by mouth, it permeates the body and crosses the brain barrier, so even taken orally it can improve circulation. Ideally it should be I.V.

One man who had a stroke at 7:30 AM refused to go to the hospital until after his wife had spoken with Dr. Stanley Jacob, which didn't happen until 6:30 PM. Starting at 7 PM the day of the stroke, she gave him one ounce of 50% DMSO in a little orange juice every 15 minutes for two hours and then every half hour for two hours. The next day, her husband was better and soon returned to normal. A substance that can stop a stroke as it's happening is something many might want in their home medicine chest. (Haley, 2000)

Angina, Heart Attacks, Injuries of the Brain and Spinal Chord

DMSO may help neutralize harmful effects on the heart and brain in medical disorders involving the head and spinal cord injury, stroke, memory dysfunction, and ischemic heart disease (Jacob, de la Torre, 2009). A 40% DMSO solution should be administered within four hours to be effective, within ninety minutes is best. in a bank. (Haley, 2000)

Infections

When combined with antibiotics, DMSO will convert bacteria which are resistant to a given antibiotic to being sensitive to that same antibiotic and probably a 80 to 90 per cent solution of DMSO will be required in order to be clinically useful (Pottz, Rampey, Benjamin,1967). DMSO has been used to transport antibiotics to hard-to-reach areas of the body with excellent results, such as the bone marrow and brain (Sanders, 1967).

DMSO can dissolve a virus protein coating, leaving the virus core unprotected with its nucleic acid exposed to the immune system. Applied topically, it alleviates the lesions that occur as a result of Herpes Zoster, shingles (Morton, 1993).

Placed into the nostrils or topically in the face, DMSO can open blocked sinuses within a few minutes and it has been used with success in patients with polyps (Marvin, 1967).

DMSO can clear up gum disease and reduce tooth decay and their pain by painting it on the involved areas.

Several books have been published on the benefits of DMSO

Keloids, Scars, Burns, Bruises

A concentration of 50 to 80% put on two or three times a day will flatten a raised scar after several months. It is of considerable value in superficial burns (Goldman, 1967) and when applied quickly to an injury, it can eliminate any bruising.

Headaches

DMSO is highly effective in vascular headaches and in muscular tension which so often goes with headaches. It may be used on hairy areas such as the scalp and it also may be used near the eyes. A 90% solution is more effective (Ogden, 1967).

Miscellaneous

DMSO in conjunction with other treatments has shown to regress cancer in a very effective way (Ayre, 1967).

Intravenous administration of DMSO markedly reduces pathological intestinal permeability while preserving the gut's absorption capacities (Wang et al, 1996). Considering that gut permeability ('leaky gut') has a fundamental role in chronic degenerative diseases, this is of great clinical importance.

DMSO also has excellent results in the skin of people afflicted with scleroderma, results which have never been observed with any other method of therapy (Scherbel et al, 1967).

Mrs. Jean Puccio of Washington, DC testified at hearings of Senator Edward Kennedy's sub-committee on health in 1980 on her recovery from scleroderma. Diagnosed in 1971, she was told that no medication would help, and that she would probably soon face a wheelchair and early death. By the time she found Dr. Jacob (through word of mouth), she told the Senators, "I was having difficulty breathing, walking, and eating". The disease "thickens the tissue and makes your skin so tight you cannot move. It was difficult for me to drive, to turn the ignition in my car or turn my body". Her dentist could not work on her for a while because she could not open her mouth. "Now I can open my mouth like anybody", she said. After her sensitized skin burned from topical application of DMSO, Dr. Jacob suggested taking it orally. "Within six months", she testified, "my condition reversed almost immediately. I can do anything anybody else can do now" (Haley, 2000).

Hopefully, this brief overview of DMSO's great capabilities has helped to illustrate how it is indeed, the cure of our times. Its uses and applications make it a very handy compound to have on your medical shelf. In pure form, the life of DMSO is indefinite, so it may be used for years.

Troubleshooting

The garlic-like body odor and taste in the mouth that some experience is attributable to a specific DMSO metabolite: dimethyl sulfide (DMS), a component of natural onion and garlic flavors (McKim, Strub, 2008). This can last for one or two days and in a small number of people, especially men, the odor can be very pungent. Drinking enough water will help diffuse the smell. Other side effects - such as stomach upset, headaches, dizziness, and sedation - are very likely related to detoxification reactions prompted by the DMSO.

Only purified and properly diluted DMSO should be used. When you dilute a pure DMSO solution, always do it in distilled water. When it is applied, the skin site as well as the applying hand should be thoroughly cleaned before application. This is of utmost importance as DMSO's properties allow contaminants to be absorbed through the skin and transported into the bloodstream.

DMSO is known to be one of the least toxic substances in biology (Parcell, 2002), so any serious side effects should come from potential contaminants or the intake of drugs that DMSO will carry into the body. Worth repeating again, DMSO and any substance dissolved in it, will penetrate the skin, the blood-brain barrier, and other parts of the body very fast.

Remember also that DMSO increases the effects of drugs like blood thinners, steroids, heart medicines, sedatives, etc. In addition to that, acetone or acid contamination of DMSO can lead to serious medical consequences. Be aware of this problem when buying unreliable DMSO. A pure DMSO solution will turn solid (like ice) in the refrigerator within 2 hours. If, when the frozen bottle is turned upside down, little rivulets of water flow through the ice, you probably possess the veterinary grade DMSO. This is a 90% concentration. Ten percent is distilled water (Morton, 1993).

Women are discouraged from using DMSO during pregnancy or breastfeeding, even though DMSO is used to preserve frozen human embryos. DMSO can interfere with liver function tests and give a false reading. That problem is easily solved by waiting a week after DMSO usage before taking the test.

Long-term use has been documented as safe. Eye damage, reported in laboratory animals, has not been confirmed. Side effects such as skin rash and itching after topical application, breaking up of blood elements after intravenous infusion, can be avoided in large part by employing more dilute solutions. Despite these side effects, DMSO is used as a preservative for blood elements and stem cells (McKim, Strub, 2008).

When DMSO is diluted with water, heat is released. The bottle will be warm to the touch. This is a temporary, harmless reaction.

Since DMSO causes dryness and scaling of the outer layer of the skin, skin diseases characterized by scaling (psoriasis) could be aggravated by the use of DMSO. But DMSO applied topically for only a few days has been useful in psoriasis. Prolonged use of DMSO for the treatment of psoriasis is not advised however, as it can worsen the condition (Engel, 1967), only DMSO taken orally is suggested.

Sulfur is an element of the earth and it is essential to life, it is among the most prevalent elements in the human body. Allergic reactions to sulfur are not possible because sulfur has no protein component. When people are 'allergic to sulfur', what they really mean is that they are allergic or sensitive mainly to certain sulfur-containing drugs or proteins, most notably sulfa antibiotics (sulfonamides) or to sulfites (preservatives used in wines and some foods), or to foods with a high sulfur content (broccoli, cauliflower, garlic, onions, etc.). Many individuals with allergies to sulfa drugs, sulfites, or high sulfur containing foods (like the author) do not experience problems taking DMSO, because apart from sulfur, DMSO bears no relation to these substances.

As always, proceed with caution, do your homework, and consult a health care provider in case of doubts.

Ref: Gabriela Segura, M.D., Sott.net, Thu, 12 May 2011 08:12 CDT

Are Multivitamins Useless?

A response by the Linus Pauling Institute to an article published in the February 2009 issue of the *Archives of Internal Medicine*.

A study published in the medical journal *Archives of Internal Medicine* (*Arch Intern Med.* 2009;169(3):294-304), which followed 161,808 women from the Women's Health Initiative over eight years, claimed to provide "convincing evidence that multivitamin use has little or no influence on the risk of common cancers, cardiovascular disease, or total mortality in postmenopausal women." This message was immediately sent around the world by the news media, leading people everywhere to believe that taking a daily multivitamin does no good and is a waste of money. Is it, really? Actually, nothing could be further from the truth.

The study was an observational study, not a randomized controlled trial. Both types of studies are called "epidemiological" or population-based studies, but there is a fundamental difference between the two of them. As its name implies, an observational study "observes" what people do, what they eat, what dietary supplements they take, how they live, and what kind of diseases they develop. Randomized controlled trials take a group of subjects and randomly assign half of them to get a specific treatment, for example, a certain pharmaceutical drug or vitamin, and the other half gets a dummy pill, or placebo. After several years, researchers assess whether those who got the actual treatment develop less disease than those who got the placebo.

Every epidemiologist will tell you that observational studies cannot establish cause-and-effect relationships; they only can observe associations. For example, a study may find that intake of a certain vitamin was associated with a lower incidence of a specific disease. Whether that vitamin was the cause for the decreased disease risk cannot be answered by an observational study. In order to answer that question, a randomized controlled trial is necessary. In other words, every epidemiologist knows that observational studies are only good enough to generate a new hypothesis, like "multivitamins might not lower risk of heart disease", but this hypothesis needs to be tested in randomized controlled trials to either prove it, establishing a cause-and-effect relationship, or refute it. Unless and until such trials have been conducted, one cannot draw any conclusions regarding causality, let alone make recommendations for the public.

Observational studies are only hypothesis-generating because they are notoriously difficult to evaluate and interpret. For example, the data are based on information collected from the participants, which is often selective and inaccurate (called "recall bias"). Behavior can change appreciably over eight years of observation. Multivitamin formulations vary considerably, and participants may have changed brands during the study. Most importantly, people who volunteer to be part of these studies are generally healthier than the average person - they are more health conscious, have a healthier diet, exercise more, etc., which can significantly affect the outcome of the study (called "healthy enrollee effect").

In the study, 41.5% of the participating women took multivitamins, and these multivitamin users were healthier than the non-users. Multivitamin users were more likely than non-users to be Caucasian, live in the Western U.S., drink moderate amounts of alcohol, smoke less, have a lower body mass index and a higher level of education, and report being physically more active and eat more fruits and vegetables and less fat. Each of these factors can strongly influence the multivitamin users' risk of disease, which makes it very difficult, if not impossible, to tease out the role of multivitamins alone. Epidemiologists use statistical models, in this case the "proportional hazards model," that they claim allows "adjusting" their data for all of these factors, but they often do not acknowledge that these statistical models are based on many assumptions and are imperfect, and are applied to incomplete and inaccurate data.

Here is the dizzying list of factors for which adjustments were made to the data in the study, quoting directly from the paper: "age; race/ethnicity; years since menopause (body mass index; education; alcohol use; smoking; general health; geographic region; physical activity, fruit and vegetable intake; percentage of energy from fat; single supplements of vitamin C, E, or calcium and any other single supplement use and stratified according to age (5-year groups), and hormone therapy trial randomization assignment or study enrollment."

Because all of these adjustments were made using imperfect data and an imperfect statistical model, they are very unlikely to reveal the true effect of multivitamins. Furthermore, despite the statisticians' best efforts to take all of these "confounding" factors into consideration, there are numerous additional factors left that haven't been discovered yet or were not measured in the study. This phenomenon is called "residual confounding" and is a major reason why observational studies can only generate hypotheses. In contrast, in randomized controlled trials subjects are randomly assigned to treatment or placebo, so all confounding factors, even the unknown ones, should be distributed equally between the two groups. That's why well-designed, randomized controlled trials are superior to observational studies and, in contrast to observational studies, can establish cause-and-effect relationships.

Given these considerations, it appears wrong for the authors of the study to conclude that it provides "convincing evidence" for multivitamins having little or no effect on cancer or cardiovascular disease risk. The evidence is far from convincing; it is suggestive at best. In addition, while endpoints like cancer, heart disease, and death are important, it is possible, for example, that a daily multivitamin helps protect against other diseases, improves immune or brain function, or promotes general health. Also, eight years of multivitamin supplementation in women over 50 years of age, as assessed in the study, may be too little too late to have a significant effect. Obviously, the data do not apply to men, because they have a different risk profile for cardiovascular diseases and hormone-dependent cancers, among many other reasons.

The reality is that most people in the U.S. have a poor diet and don't come close to consuming the recommended nine servings of fruit and vegetables every day. As a consequence, high percentages of the U.S. population do not meet the recommended dietary allowances — set by the U.S. Institute of Medicine — for many vitamins and essential minerals, including vitamins A, C, E, and K, folic acid, zinc, magnesium, and calcium. For example, data from the National Health and Nutrition Examination Survey indicate that over 90% of the population doesn't meet the recommended dietary intake for vitamin E, over 40% for vitamin A, 30% for vitamin C, and 50% for magnesium. And evidence is accumulating that most people in the U.S. are vitamin D deficient.

Given the reality that people will not improve their diet and often cannot afford to buy more fruits and vegetables, the next best thing and most cost-effective solution is to take a multivitamin. Despite the cynics' assertion that "popping vitamins is a waste of money," taking a daily multivitamin costs less than 10 cents a day. Even certain principals of the Women's Health Initiative acknowledge that "the research doesn't mean multivitamins are useless. Multivitamins may still be useful as a form of [health] insurance for people with poor eating habits." And let's not fool ourselves, that's the large majority of the people in this country!

https://www.npscript.com/dougcaporrino/vita-vitamin-multi-vitamin/OL0245PAR#undefined2

Calcium Myths

People generally think that they need calcium in their diet (and they are right), but they also think that they need *a lot* of calcium and that milk is the only way to get enough.

There are many reasons why you might want to consider removing milk and milk products from your diet. Studies are starting to show just what kind of negative impact our love affair with the cow has on our health and even on our bones. When I suggest to people that they stop milk and any dairy, I can almost guarantee that the next thing out of their mouths is, "yes, but where do I get my calcium?" Their response speaks to the power, effectiveness, and tragedy (for our health) of advertising and the Great Milk Lobby.

My answer to their question of where do you get enough calcium is to ask another question: "Where do cows, moose, and even elephants (who all have very strong bones) get their calcium if all they eat is grass?"

Foods high in calcium

While you might think that the only good source of calcium is milk, there are others. Yes, milk does contain calcium (1 cup has 296 mg of calcium), but milk is, by far, not the only good source of calcium. Take a look at these other foods:

- Sesame seeds (1 cup = 702 mg)
- Flax seeds (1 cup = 416 mg)
- Cabbage (1 cup = 380 mg)

- Collard greens (1 cup = 266 mg)
- Spinach (1 cup = 245 mg)
- Orange (1 cup = 104 mg)
- Kale (1 cup = 94 mg)
- Broccoli (1 cup = 62 mg)

High Milk Intake Associated with Higher Rates of Death (Mortality) & Fractures:

From a 2014 ***British Medical Journal (BMJ)*** study titled: "Milk intake and risk of mortality and fractures in women and men: cohort studies" – summary excerpts: "Objective: To examine whether high milk consumption is associated with mortality and fractures in women and men… Participants: Two large Swedish cohorts, one with 61,433 women… and one with 45,339 men… **Conclusions: High milk intake was associated with higher mortality in one cohort of women and in another cohort of men, and with higher fracture incidence in women…**"

Reference: "Milk intake and risk of mortality and fractures in women and men: cohort studies", BMJ 2014; 349; http://www.bmj.com/content/349/bmj.g6015

A 2014 news report: "**Three glasses of milk a day can lead to early death, warn scientists**. Drinking three glasses of milk **doubles the risk of early death** and does not prevent broken bones, new research has shown…

A study that tracked 61,000 women and 45,000 men for 20 years found there was no reduction in broken bones for those who consumed the most milk…"

Source: http://www.telegraph.co.uk/news/health/news/11193329/Three-glasses-of-milk-a-day-can-lead-to-early-death-warn-scientists.html

In a journal of the *American Medical Association,* medical doctors Ludwig & Willett state: "**Humans have no nutritional requirement for animal milk… many populations throughout the world today**

consume little or no milk... bone fracture rates tend to be lower in countries that do not consume milk compared with those that do. Moreover, milk consumption does not protect against fracture in adults, according to recent meta-analysis."

Reference: "Three Daily Servings of Reduced-Fat Milk. An Evidence-Based Recommendation?" JAMA Pediatrics, 2013;167(9):788-789; at https://jamanetwork.com/journals/jamapediatrics/article-abstract/1704826

Dairy Milk Consumption Association with Higher Rates of Cancer:

From an article titled "Do dairy products cause cancer?" by The Physicians Committee for Responsible Medicine: "**Recent scientific studies have suggested that dairy products may be linked to increased risk for prostate cancer, testicular cancer, and possibly for ovarian and breast cancers.**

Prostate cancer has been linked to dairy products in several studies. In Harvard's Physicians Health Study, including more than 20,000 male physicians, **those who consumed more than two dairy servings daily had a 34% higher risk of developing prostate cancer** than men who consumed little or no dairy products. Several other studies have shown much the same thing...

A recent analysis of studies examining a relationship between dairy product consumption and ovarian cancer risk found that for every 10 grams of lactose consumed (the amount in one glass of milk), ovarian cancer risk increased by 13 percent..."

Reference: http://www.pcrm.org/health/cancer-resources/ask/ask-the-expert-dairy-products

"Prostate Cancer and Organic Milk vs. Almond Milk"

This recent study… controlling for as many factors as possible by just isolating prostate cancer cells out of the body in a petri dish, and dripping cow milk on them directly. They chose organic cows' milk because they wanted to exclude the effect of added hormones, and just test the effect of all the growth and sex hormones found naturally in all milk.

They found that "**cow's milk stimulated the growth of [human] prostate cancer cells in each of 14 separate experiments,** producing an average increase in [cancer] growth rate of over 30%. In contrast, almond milk suppressed the growth of these cancer cells by over 30%." …

The latest meta-analysis of all the best case control studies ever done on the matter concludes that milk consumption is a risk factor for prostate cancer. And the latest meta-analysis of all the best cohort studies ever done also concludes that **milk consumption is a risk factor for prostate cancer.** An even newer study suggests that milk intake during adolescence may be particularly risky in terms of potentially setting one up for cancer later in life."

Clip: https://www.youtube.com/watch?v=qAnD9XKI7J4
Text: https://nutritionfacts.org/video/prostate-cancer-and-organic-milk-vs-almond-milk/

There are countless studies done on the negative effects of dairy and yet we are still fed a steady stream if "Got Milk" ads.

The bottom line is "Why Guess, Test", to see exactly what your nutrient depletions are and then correct them through proper menu or supplementation.

Vitamin E Does Not Cause Prostate Cancer

I've talked about how hysteria sells news. I also specifically mentioned a recent study that "proved" that "Vitamin Pills Are Useless._Or at least that's what the mainstream media wanted you to believe.

There was another SELECT Study on Vitamin E and prostate cancer. Absurdly, it has concluded that vitamin E causes prostate cancer.

Vitamin E causes prostate cancer????

On October 12th, the researchers conducting the *Selenium and Vitamin E Cancer Prevention Trial* (aka the SELECT Study) published the results of their eight year investigation (the study actually ran from 2001 to 2008) by announcing that vitamin E supplementation not only does not help prevent prostate cancer; it actually increases your risk of getting it — substantially.

Wow!

Specifically, the study found that men over 50 who take 400 IU of vitamin E a day actually demonstrate a 17 percent increased risk of getting prostate cancer, which is statistically significant — particularly when calculated over a population of millions of men taking dedicated supplements and/or multivitamins with large doses of vitamin E. Even worse, the researchers found that vitamin E's negative effects can continue even after men stop taking the supplement. In other words, according to the study, if you're a man and you've been taking vitamin E for years and you stop now that you've read the report, you're still screwed!

In summary, according to the researchers, "There just doesn't seem to be a reason to be taking vitamin E if you are a man over 55 or 60." Also, according to Eric Klein, one of the study's authors, the study underscores "the importance of large-scale, population-based, randomized trials to accurately measure the benefit or harm of micronutrients such as diet supplements."

Dr. Ian Thompson, another one of the study's authors, may have added the pièce de résistance when, as a point of reference, he compared the vitamin E study to a study on beta-carotene that took place several years ago, stating that researchers once had high hopes that beta-carotene, a vitamin A precursor that is fat-soluble like vitamin E, might prevent lung cancer. But like vitamin E and prostate cancer, it had the opposite effect.

Wow again!

Enough of the nonsense

In truth, there is no surprise in these results. There is no "Wow" factor here.

Currently, one of the largest cancer studies in US history is underway: The Selenium and Vitamin E Cancer Prevention Trial (SELECT). The study is taking place in the United States, Puerto Rico, and Canada. Its goal is to find out if taking selenium and/or vitamin E supplements can prevent prostate cancer in men age 50 or older. The SELECT trial is expected to stop recruiting patients in May 2006. The study will continue for 7 years after the last man has enrolled, meaning that each man will participate for 7 years or more, depending on when he joins the study. More than 400 sites in the United States, Puerto Rico, and Canada are taking part in the study. Over 32,000 men will participate in SELECT. Sounds impressive, yes?

Well here's the catch.

- The vitamin E they're using is dl-alpha-tocopherol — the synthetic isolate form of vitamin E, the least effective form possible.

On the other hand, the selenium they're using is l-selenomethionine, (Selen o meth ion nine) which is an organic, highly useable form of selenium. The study gets points for that.

But based on the forms of antioxidants being used, the results of the study are highly predictable even before it starts.

- Selenium helps
- Vitamin E does not
- There is little synergistic effect from the use of selenium and Vitamin E together.

Well, here it is seven and a half years later (the study finished early), and except for the results on selenium by itself, the analysis was spot on. And as for selenium, the result doesn't necessarily mean what the study says it does, but we'll have to save that discussion for another time.

Let's take a closer look at the details of the study to pick up some of the nuances of its stupidity.

We can begin with a little lesson in the history and chemical makeup of vitamin E.

What is vitamin E

As the old saying goes, you can't tell the players without a scorecard. So, let's take a look at vitamin E and define what we're talking about.

When most people think of vitamin E, they think of alpha-tocopherol — after all, that's the chemical name listed on your vitamin bottle. But the surprising truth is that vitamin E is not a single substance. It is actually a complex of at least eight compounds. There are four tocopherols and four tocotrienols that are all identified as having vitamin E activity.

Although natural health practitioners had been proclaiming the benefits of an unidentified substance in certain oils — especially wheat germ oil — for decades, it was not until 1922 that vitamin E was first "discovered," and not until 1936 that tocopherols were actually isolated by researchers. Amazingly, it wasn't until 1968, almost 50 years after first being discovered, that the Food and Nutrition Board of the US National Research Council actually acknowledged that vitamin E is an essential nutrient for humans

As it turns out, alpha-tocopherol is the form of vitamin E that is the most absorbable, the most prevalent, and the most active in the human body. Thus, scientists just assumed it was the most important — thus making it the measure for vitamin E supplementation. Unfortunately:

- Just because it's the most prevalent and most active, doesn't necessarily make it the most important for your health.
    - More recent studies have found that gamma-tocopherol may be more important, more essential. Gamma tocopherol plays an extremely important role defending against systemic inflammation caused by reactive nitrogen oxide compounds such as nitrogen dioxide and peroxynitrite — both of which are major components of automobile exhaust and cigarette smoke. Gamma-tocopherol may also protect against Alzheimer's disease and prostate cancer — and most particularly relevant, especially when considering the results of the SELECT Study, there is the study that found that gamma-tocopherol inhibits cell proliferation and DNA synthesis in prostate cancer cells, whereas alpha-tocopherol does not.
    - As for tocotrienols, there is abundant research that indicates that all four tocotrienols may be more important to your health and longevity than alpha-tocopherol — in fact, demonstrating 40-60 times the antioxidant activity.
    - But most significant of all, studies now indicate that supplementing with high doses of alpha-tocopherol may decrease the body's ability to absorb gamma-tocopherol, while at the same time, reducing the effects of tocotrienols that you do absorb — again, an important consideration when evaluating the results of the SELECT Study.

The bottom line is that back in the early 1900's, scientists didn't know about the importance of all the other components of vitamin E. In the end, they made a logical but incorrect assumption: if alpha-tocopherol is the most prevalent form of vitamin E in the body, it must be the most important component and, therefore, the only one worth measuring. Thus, was born the standard of measuring vitamin E by its alpha-tocopherol content — which wouldn't necessarily be a problem if it weren't for the economics of manufacturing supplements. Quite simply, it's much cheaper to just add one component to a supplement as opposed to eight. Yes, you could use a complete oil extract of all vitamin E components from a natural oil and just "list" its vitamin E content by measuring the alpha-tocopherol levels, but that would be so much more expensive than using just alpha-tocopherol — particularly if you could synthesize it from something much less expensive than natural vegetable oils. (And in fact, only a small handful of manufacturers cared enough to do it right.)

In any case, thus was born synthetic alpha-tocopherol made from petroleum, turpentine, sugar, and artificial preservatives. Yum!

Natural VS synthetic alpha-tocopherol

Natural alpha-tocopherol, as found in foods and naturally sourced supplements, is known as d-alpha-tocopherol, whereas synthetic alpha-tocopherol, created in a laboratory, is known as dl-alpha-tocopherol. What's the difference?

Most supplement manufacturers (other than a handful of purists) would tell you there is none. Your doctor would tell you there is none. And most scientists, including the researchers running the SELECT Study, it would seem, would tell you there is none.

But they are wrong! There is a world of difference — recognized by those scientists who keep up-to-date on vitamin research, as well as anyone who actually understands holistic health.

How can there be such a difference of opinion?

The problem is that both natural and synthetic vitamin E have the same chemical formula: And that similarity is enough for most scientists and today's FDA. But, in fact, the way those atoms are arranged, although similar, varies between natural and synthetic versions. In truth, there are seven synthetic variations of alpha tocopherol (not one of which can be found in nature), and they are all arranged in various mirror images to the natural form in what is known as stereoisomers.

It should be noted that the alpha-tocopherol used in the SELECT Study was identified as "all-racemic alpha-tocopherol acetate," which means it was a mixture of all eight stereoisomers. The important thing to understand about this mixture is that only one alpha-tocopherol molecule in eight is in the natural RRR-alpha-tocopherol form. That's means only 12.5% of the total alpha-tocopherol ingested in the study was in the natural form. 87.5% was synthetic!

But the question is: why should it matter? If the molecules contain the exact same atoms and are virtually identical, other than certain groupings within the molecule being mirror images of each other, what difference does it make? After all, nutrition experts don't seem to care, allowing all variations (synthetic and natural) to be used interchangeably on labels. And in fact, it's impossible to notice any visual difference between the stereoisomers,

There is no argument among scientists that actually keep up on the research that the natural d-alpha-tocopherol is more potent gram for gram than the synthetic dl-alpha tocopherol. In fact, many years ago, the natural form was officially recognized by the FDA, the World Health Organization, and the United States Pharmacopoeia as 36% more potent than the synthetic. But even at that, government sources might be understating the issue. A study done out of the Steacie Institute for Molecular Sciences, through the National Research Council of Canada, concluded that natural d-alpha-tocopherol is, in fact, twice as bioavailable as the synthetic form. Even more suggestive is a study done with pregnant women out of the Eastman Center for Nutrition Research at the James H Quillen College of Medicine (part of East Tennessee State University). Researchers there found that natural d-alpha tocopherol passed through the placentas of the pregnant women to their babies three times more efficiently than did the synthetic.

But that doesn't even tell the whole story. The FDA allows blended natural/synthetic dl-alpha-tocopherol to be labeled as "Natural E" even though it may contain as little as 5% natural alpha-tocopherol. As a result, oftentimes, even when you think you are buying 100% Natural E, you are not! It very well may be 95% synthetic. 100% natural vitamin E, when you actually get it, may be as much as 500% more effective than the synthetic — or the misleadingly labeled "natural."

Conclusion

Running a study on synthetic vitamin E isolate and then broadcasting the negative results as an indictment of "all" forms of vitamin E — especially considering that the scientific community has already acknowledged the inferiority of dl-alpha-tocopherol — is like running a study on the quality of fake Rolex watches and coming to the conclusion, based on that study, that all Rolex watches are junk...and then promoting those results to the gullible world press, desperate for any outrageous headline that can sell papers or boost ratings. It is false logic. It is bad advice. It is unethical. And it is ultimately dangerous in that it will encourage many people to make a bad health choice when it comes to supplementation with vitamin E.

If you supplement with vitamin E, which is probably a good idea despite the study, make sure you use only the all-natural form, and make sure it's a complete vitamin E complex with all four tocopherols and all four tocotrienols. (If the label doesn't specifically say that the supplement contains all eight naturally occurring Vitamin E compounds, then it doesn't. As I've already discussed, when it comes to vitamin E, the word "natural" by itself doesn't mean much.)

If you ever see another study again slamming vitamin E, check first to see if it was done using all natural, full-complex E. If not, you can throw the study in the trash where it belongs.

And if you opt for a multivitamin supplement, make sure you choose one that is food formed, or "grown" — not packed with synthetics and isolates.

The Benefits of Epsom Salts

Bath salts offer many added benefits to a regular bath.

These special salts aid in the **healing of dry skin** by opening the pores to **purify the skin, cleansing away dirt, sweat and toxins**.

The addition of salts to a bath can also in improving the skin's resistance to allergic factors, soothes insect bites, minor rashes and even calluses. Also, bath salt has been proven effective in treating some serious cases that are induced by pathogenic factors like athlete's foot, psoriasis and eczema.

Aromatherapy bath salts, or simply salts infused with essential oils, offer the added benefit of aromatherapy. Pleasant scents have been shown to promote relaxation. And depending on the type of essential oils used, an aromatherapy bath salt can also provide other healing properties.

One popular bath salt is **Epsom Salt** which is good for exfoliation. But that's not the only benefit that you can achieve by using Epsom salt.

A lot of people have been found to suffer from **magnesium deficiency**. This nutrient deficiency accounts for the high rates of heart disease, stroke, osteoporosis, arthritis, digestive ailments, stress-related illnesses, chronic fatigue and other diseases.

Recent studies show

Studies show that magnesium isn't easily absorbed by ingestion of foods, drugs or supplements. However, soaking in a bath with Epsom salt has shown to give a great magnesium boost.

Epsom salts known scientifically as hydrated magnesium sulfate, is rich in both magnesium and sulfate, both of which can be poorly absorbed through the stomach but are easily absorbed through the skin.

Sulfates also play an important role in the body as they help with the formation of brain tissue, joint proteins and proteins that line the walls of the digestive tract. Sulfates also help detoxify the body.

Epsom salt baths are also part of cancer treatment programs. Epsom salt baths **help neutralize toxins** by assisting the body's elimination of them through the skin as well as relieving tired nerves.

Along with this bath, drinking diaphoretic teas, which induce perspiration, like elder, yarrow, peppermint, boneset or ginger also helps eliminate toxins. Pyrogens, which raise body temperature, are also released which helps enhance resistance, strengthen the immune system and stimulate phagocytosis, which helps get rid of harmful bacteria. A hot Epsom salt bath is also known to increase heart rate, respiration, metabolism and circulation.

Adding essential oils to an Epsom salt bath also adds the benefits of aromatherapy. Lavender oils is a favorite for most people, with tangerine and rosemary also being highly recommended, especially for morning baths. These three essential oils possess anticancer activity and the Epsom salt can be a simple but effective way to employ the aromatics.

To reap all the benefits from your aromatherapy bath salt-enhanced bath simply add 2 cups of Epsom salt and 10 to 20 drops of your choice of essential oil to a tub of hot water (106 to 108 degrees Fahrenheit). Soak in the bath until your body reaches 101 degrees, which should take around 15 to 20 minutes.

Warnings

However, Epsom salt baths aren't for everyone. It's not recommended for anyone with low blood cell count, pregnant women and people suffering from several other health concerns. Before going through a regular routine of using Epsom salt baths, do consult with your doctor.

Reasons Not to Get the Flu Shot

According to the Centers for Disease Control and Prevention's (CDC) *Morbidity and Mortality Weekly Report* published September 19th, 58.9 percent of children ages 6 months to 17 years got the flu vaccine during the 2013-2014 flu season along with 42.2 percent of adults 18 years and older—an estimated 143.2 million total—all under the assumption that they were doing something good for themselves, their families, and their communities. After all, by protecting yourself from the flu you're protecting those around you, right?

Unfortunately, this may not be the case. **A growing body of evidence is starting to surface that supports the inefficacy and possible dangers of the flu vaccine.** One quick search on the Internet will take you to some credible and informative websites on the topic. Yet still, most Americans choose to take the "safe" stance on flu vaccination and follow the advice of physicians and the CDC. If you're one of the estimated 143.2 million Americans that gets vaccinated, sadly, this may wind up doing you more harm than good. Below are three good reasons why you might want to reconsider getting the flu shot.

1. **There is little proof the flu vaccine is effective.**
   - Given that there are over 200 viruses that cause influenza and influenza-like illnesses and **there is no way to predict exactly which strain will hit each year, researchers make an educated guess** and the vaccine manufacturers create

a vaccine based on this guess. This means that **when the researchers guess wrongly, millions of Americans get vaccinated against the wrong flu strain**.

- The British Medical Journal (BMJ) researched 259 studies on influenza vaccine efficacy and concluded that **vaccine industry and government sponsored studies were of considerably lower quality and more in favor of vaccination**. That is, **the higher the quality** and the more independently resourced, **the less likely the study was to support vaccination**. Another research article published by Cochrane Summaries in March 2014 concluded that "**influenza vaccines have a very modest effect in reducing influenza symptoms**."
- Simply read the CDC's own page on influenza vaccine effectiveness. Statements such as the following leave much to be questioned: "**How well the flu vaccine works** (or its ability to prevent flu illness) **can range widely** from season to season." Or, "Results of studies that assess how well a flu vaccine works can vary based on study design, outcome(s) measured, population studied and the season in which the vaccine was studied. **These differences can make it difficult to compare one study's results with another's**."

2. **Vaccines contain harmful adjuvants and preservatives, and possibly viral proteins**.
   - The CDC itself has reported that **brain inflammation and death are known side effects of every vaccine**. What most people don't take into consideration is that conditions such as autism, ADHD and learning disabilities are manifestations of an inflamed brain. Below is a list of **ingredients found in flu vaccines**:
     - **Aluminum compounds**: a neurotoxin associated with Alzheimer's and dementia
     - **Ammonium sulfate**: attributed to respiratory toxicity
     - **Beta-Propiolactdone**: a chemical linked to malignant lymphatic tumors in animals

        - **Ethyl mercury (thimerosal)**: a neurotoxin that has been associated with autism, dyslexia, mental retardation and seizures
        - **Formaldehyde**: a known carcinogen, neurotoxin, and gene disruptor
        - **Monosodium glutamate**: a preservative associated with delayed learning, and behavioral and reproductive disorders
        - **Oxtoxinol-9**: a vaginal spermicide
        - **Phenol**: a toxin that is disruptive to the cardiovascular, nervous, reproductive and respiratory systems
        - **Polysorbate 80**: a synthetic compound that may cause anaphylactic shock and is a known carcinogen in animals
    - **Flu vaccines may contain numerous viral proteins from chick embryos.** Pharmaceutical companies commonly use chick embryos to culture flu strains. Fertilized chicken eggs (humans eat *un*fertilized eggs) are susceptible to a wide variety of viruses and contain active biologic ingredients that may be harmful to humans, such as tiny proteins associated with neurological disorders and oncogenes—genes that transform normal cells into cancerous ones.

3. **Influenza is not a serious threat.**
    - How many people do you know have died from having the flu? Mostly likely none. In 2005 Peter Doshi—Assistant Professor at the University of Maryland School of Pharmacy and Associate Editor of BMJ (British Medical Journal)—wrote an article exposing how the CDC spins its death by "pneumonia and influenza" statistics. According to the CDC's National Center for Health Statistics (NCHS), "influenza and pneumonia" took 62,034 lives in 2001—61,777 of which were attributed to pneumonia and 257 to flu. In **only 18 cases was flu virus positively identified.**
    - According to the CDC: "Over a period of 30 years, between 1976 and 2006, estimates of flu-associated deaths in the United States range from a low of about 3,000 to a high

of about 49,000 people." The range is so great because **the tests to diagnose an influenza virus from one of the 150-200 pathogens that produce flu-like symptoms are not sensitive enough to decipher the difference.**

- The CDC uses respiratory and circulatory (R&C) deaths as "the primary outcome in its mortality modeling because R&C deaths provide an estimate of deaths that include secondary respiratory or cardiac complications that follow influenza." It admits, though, that "**only 2.1% of all respiratory and circulatory deaths were influenza-related**." In addition, a 2010 study published in the International Journal of Medicine concluded that **the flu vaccine contributes to cardiovascular inflammation, and thus may increase the risk of heart attack.**
- The CDC uses pneumonia and influenza (P&I) deaths as a secondary mortality model, yet it again admits that "**only 8.5% of all pneumonia and influenza deaths were influenza-related**."

Remember, getting the flu during the fall and winter months is not inevitable just because health professionals propose this time to be "flu season." Frequent hand washing with regular soap (not anti-bacterial) and a healthy lifestyle are far better and safer ways to prevent the onset of the flu than any pharmaceutical medication or vaccine on the market. If you're concerned about getting the flu, speak with a physician that has a solid knowledge of natural ways to keep it at bay.

References:

"Flu Vaccination Coverage, United States, 2013-14 Influenza Season." *Centers for Disease Control and Prevention.* n.d. Web. n.p.

Demicheli V, Jefferson T, Al-Ansary LA, Ferroni E, Rivetti A, Di Pietrantonj C. Vaccines for preventing influenza in healthy adults. Cochrane Database of Systematic Reviews 2014, Issue 3. Art. No.: CD001269. DOI: 10.1002/14651858.CD001269.pub5

BMJ 2009;338: b354 doi:10.1136/bmj. b354

Null, Gary PhD, and Gale, Richard. A New Flu Season of Pain, Profit, and Politics. *GreenMedInfo*. Web. 22 Nov 2013.

"Vaccine Effectiveness—How Well Does the Flu Vaccine Work?" *Centers for Disease Control and Prevention*. n.d. Web. n.p.

J Intern Med. 2011 Jan;269(1):118-25. doi: 10.1111/j.1365-2796.2010.02285.x. Epub. 2010 Oct 22.

BMJ 2005; 331:1412

"Estimating Seasonal Influenza-Associated Deaths in the United States: CDC Study Confirms Variability of Flu." *Centers for Disease Control and Prevention*. n.d. Web. n.p.

Brogan, Kelly MD. A Shot Never Worth Taking: The Flu Vaccine." *International Medical Council on Vaccination*. Web. 27 Nov 2013.

TEFLON, PFC, PTFE and Your Health

The next time you pick up that Teflon coated nonstick cooking pan or pot or think about getting your carpet treated to make it waterproof, think again. Perflourinated chemicals or PFC as they are called is the group of chemicals that makes them so durable and tough. While these properties may make their use seem a very attractive choice it is not at all a healthy idea. Let's see how PFC s can have an adverse impact your health.

What are perfluorinated chemicals?

Organic compounds consist of chains made up of groups of carbon and hydrogen atoms to which one or more functional groups are attached. Very simply perflourinated chemicals are long chained organic compounds where fluorine atoms take the place of hydrogen atoms in the carbon chains. Teflon is an example of a PFC.

The fluorine and carbon bond is much stronger than a carbon and hydrogen bond which gives these chemicals their unique properties and uses. They are tough, water proof, resist stains and are chemically very inert. They make durable coating for cooking pans, make paints scratch proof and make carpets, clothes and furniture water resistant. They are used for fighting fires where water cannot be used. They are not affected by agents such as acids and oxidants which can react with most other chemicals.

PFC an environmental hazard:

Perfluorinated chemicals being very stable do not break down easily and accumulate in the environment. They are easily carried over long distances by air, water and ocean currents. They get into the bodies of animals through the respiratory system or through food and thus accumulate in the food chain.

Accumulation of PFC in our body:

Perflourinated chemicals get into our body when we eat food contaminated with PFC or by consuming meat of animals that have been exposed to PFC. Degradation of cooking pans and food wraps are another source of contamination. Consumption of contaminated fish and milk products and inhalation of PFC dust are also responsible for human exposure. Unfortunately, small children are the most affected by PFC dust inhalation.

The research on two compounds called PFOA and PFOS which are the ones widely studied has established that PFC exposure is higher in advanced countries and the highest in the US probably due to the higher use of these chemicals and higher consumption of processed food. These chemicals bind to albumin in our blood and are also excreted in breast milk. They have a long half-life of 4 to 5 years which means that they don't leave our bodies easily. This has been confirmed by research on people who work in industries which manufacture PFC.

Adverse health effects of PFC:

The health problems caused by PFC are still under study. Most studies have been done on animals and these indicate serious health hazards:

- **Liver damage:** Liver enlargement has been noticed in animals that were exposed to high dosages of PFC.
- **Impact on growth and development:** Animal studies have confirmed that PFC causes higher number of neonatal deaths and interferes with the development and growth of the offspring. It has also been shown to affect the functioning of the thyroid hormone in humans.
- **Impact on reproductive hormones:** Animal studies have confirmed that PFC affects the levels of testosterone and also causes tumors and other abnormalities.
- **Infertility:** Blood tests on women who took longer than average to conceive have shown a higher than average level of PFC. Tests have also indicated that women with increased serum PFC content are also likely to have irregular menstrual cycles. In men PFC has been linked to inferior semen quality and lower sperm counts.
- **Cancer:** Though the results are not very conclusive due to the limited sample size, it has been found in one study that workers in PFC manufacturing units had higher incidence of bladder cancer. A higher incidence of prostate cancer was noticed in workers who have worked longer in such units.
- **Effects on the immune system:** PFC has been shown to make changes in the immune system in mice which may make the body more sensitive to allergens and less effective in combating pathogens.
- **Cholesterol:** PFC is suspected to play a role in increase in bad cholesterol in humans.

To reduce your exposure to PFC:

- Reduce the use of commercially packed food which could be packed in containers that have a coating of PFC to prevent the oil or fats from soaking into the packing. French fries and pizzas packed in boxes are examples of foods that could have PFC coating in the wrappings.

- Make sure that you don't buy furniture and furnishings such as carpets which are treated with PFC. Also avoid getting these items stain or dirt proofed as the chemicals used for doing this often contains PFC.
- Take care when you buy clothes, check for Teflon in the labels and pay special attention if the garment in question is coated for water or stain resistance.
- Put your safety ahead of convenience. Use alternatives instead of Teflon coated or other nonstick cookware.
- Check the ingredients of the cosmetics you use for chemicals with names like "fluoro".

Several governments and agencies have recognized the dangers of perfluorinated chemicals and are seeking to either ban their use in certain products or discourage their use. The European Union and Canada have taken the lead in regulating the use of PFC. Perfluorinated chemicals are also the subject of some global treaties which aim at restricting their use.

Top 10 Fitness Myths

If your workout buddy says sit-ups help tone your tummy and get rid of the spare tire, she must know, right? Well, maybe not. Your friend's top workout moves could lead to injuries, not a loss of inches from your waistline.

"People create beliefs based on partial truths and pass them on as law,"

Plus, we all want to believe in fast fitness fixes.

"People give full credence to one 'magical' fix. In reality, it's a combination of things – better sleep, eating less, working out more, drinking plenty of water – that yields true results."

Chances are you've fallen for one or more of the following 10 fitness myths. Who hasn't?

Fitness Myth #1: No pain, no gain. If you haven't worked out in a while – or you're trying a new kind of workout plan – you'll probably be sore the next day. Believe it or not, that's a good thing.

These aches are called "delayed onset muscle soreness,

It means that the workout created "good" micro-tears in the muscles, which heal on their own and make you stronger.

But how can you tell the difference between soreness and muscle damage?

"If soreness lasts more than 48 hours, you've overdone it," "This level of muscle damage can take six weeks to heal."

Fitness Myth #2: You need to break a sweat for exercise to work. Many women think, *If I'm not dripping with sweat, I'm not working hard enough.*

But sweat isn't a good indicator of how hard you're working. That's because too many factors affect perspiration. "People sweat at different rates."

Plus, weather – the temperature and humidity – makes a difference too.

A better measure of effort is your heart rate - or the Borg Rating of Perceived Exertion (RPE), which ranks how hard you *feel* your body is working.

It's based on several physical sensations, including increased heart and breathing rates and muscle fatigue. On a basic RPE scale, zero is "no effort," such as sitting on a couch, and 10 is "exhaustion."

The recommended RPE for most people is usually 3 (moderate) to 5 (strong), according to the American Council of Exercise.

Even easier? The talk test, which is recommended by the Centers for Disease Control and Prevention (CDC). During moderate-intensity exercise, you should be able to speak but not sing.

Fitness Myth #3: Sit-ups blast belly fat. If you do 100 crunches, you'd expect to burn major belly fat. Unfortunately, your body just doesn't work that way.

There's no direct metabolic connection between abdominal muscles and the fat cells surrounding them,

The body pulls fat from all over. It's sent to the liver to be converted into fatty acids, which travel back to your muscles as fuel,

That means any fat your body recruits for energy when you're doing repeated sit-ups could come from the arms, thighs, butt and tummy.

So, what's the secret to shedding belly fat – or any fat? Follow a balanced program of cardio and strength training, plus eat a healthy diet.

But don't give up the crunches. Even if you're not losing tummy fat, an ab workout plan helps tone and suck in that flabby belly, giving the appearance of a slimmer waist.

Plus, toning happens faster than weight loss. It's one of the speediest ways to see changes in your body.

Fitness Myth #4: A short workout is a waste of time. Who wants to spend hours pounding a treadmill? You don't have to. Shorter workouts can get you in the best shape of your life and still allow time for work, raising kids and cuddle time with your honey.

Mini-workouts – 10 minutes three times a day – are just as effective as a continuous 30-minute workout, according to the American College of Sports Medicine.

But there's a catch: You have to work harder.

"The key to spending less time in the gym is to keep the intensity high,"

How? revving your heart rate with intervals, plyometrics (explosive movements, like jumping) and a variety of exercises.

Fitness Myth #5: If I work out, I can eat what I want. True, exercise burns calories, but not enough to make up for a daily French fry habit.

Weight loss requires burning more calories than you take in. It's just easier (not to mention smarter) to control what you take in.

For example, running a mile is hard, yet it only burns 100 calories. And a grueling 3-mile run (300 calories used) won't make up for a large 500-calorie packet of fries.

But there's good news: Great workouts can help balance an occasional high-calorie splurge.

"Exercise allows you to eat some of the things you crave, but you still have to eat well [regularly] to balance your diet,"

Fitness Myth #6: Lifting weights is only for men. Sure, a weight room can be intimidating for women, but it's not a men-only zone. Lifting weights can help women tone up, slim down and still keep their girlish figures.

Don't worry about getting muscle-bound: Women aren't wired to build bulky muscles because they don't produce enough testosterone. (Yes, women make the male hormone too.) Weight-lifting can help women develop sleek muscle, which improves body shape and fitness. Plus, resistance training increases a woman's bone density and allows more efficient fat burning. It also improves posture, muscle tone, endurance and strength.

Fitness Myth #7: Morning is the best time to work out. There's no single perfect time to get in those workout moves. It depends on you. If you constantly hit the snooze button to postpone a 5 a.m. workout, rethink your goals.

The best time of day to exercise is whenever you'll actually do it. That could mean lunchtime, after work or later in the evening when the kids are in bed.

"If working out in the evening replaces sitting on the couch, watching TV and eating junk food, do it,

For many people, a morning workout plan is best because they're less likely to be distracted later on.

"As the day goes on, excuses tend to pile up and eventually workouts are skipped, altogether, So, pick a time when you have the most energy, need the stress release or have the best chance of making exercise a habit.

Fitness Myth #8: If the scale hasn't budged, you're not making progress. Don't be a slave to the scale. A pound is a pound, whether it's made up of muscle, fat or feathers.

Density, not weight, is what matters.

"Picture a pound of lean ground hamburger you buy at the grocery store – that's what a pound of muscle looks like,

Double that, and you have a good idea of how big a pound of fat is.

Muscle is more compact than fat, so it takes up less space in your body. Which explains why the scale may not budge, even as your belt gets looser and clothes fit better.

Fitness Myth #9: Exercise doesn't help shed pounds, so why bother? Most of us want to drop a few pounds, but weight loss shouldn't be the only reason to get moving.

In fact, if you stopped focusing on the scale and how your body looks, you might notice that exercise makes you feel better.

A regular dose of cardio, strength-training, flexibility and balance exercises fights stress and improves brain and nervous system function.

Fitness Myth #10: A sports drink is a workout must-have. Staying hydrated during a workout is important, but unless you'll be sweating it out for 90 minutes or more, don't drink anything but water.

The body's not working so hard that it'll run out of electrolytes or glucose, so a sports drink will only add unnecessary calories to your diet. If you want to add electrolytes just put a pinch of Himalayan salt in your water.

What is Really in Laundry Detergent?

Laundry detergent, according to many researchers, is a danger to the environment and to the health of every person who uses it. To most people, such claims come across like an exaggerated conspiracy theory. Some skeptics even laugh at such notions and ask, if laundry detergent is so dangerous, why aren't men, women and children, getting violently sick every time they put on freshly washed clothes.

In the book, **"Never Be Sick Again" by Raymond Francis**, an MIT trained scientist, tells how he brought himself back from the brink of death, and since then, countless other individuals as well, by following and teaching his new model of human health and sickness.

He says, **there is only one disease**: cellular malfunction. It, in turn, manifests in countless symptoms, that are incorrectly labeled as various diseases and disorders, both large and small — for instance, everything from cancer to the common cold.

He tells us there are only two possible causes of cellular malfunction: deficiency and toxins. Symptoms (what we currently think of as illnesses), originate due to the lack of something our cells need (certain nutrients), or because they are being adversely affected my unnatural poisons. The poisons are all around us in our synthetic environment.

They are extremely prevalent in our personal care products, including (and especially) in our laundry detergents. Francis says that the thing to remember about these chemical poisons is that their effects are cumulative. Just as one cigarette is not going to kill you, exposure to toxins, over the years, clog up your body's detoxification abilities and can drastically affect your immune system until your life is in jeopardy.

Moreover, it is not uncommon for some individuals to develop heightened sensitivities to certain chemicals in laundry products that will create profoundly negative health consequences requiring emergency hospitalization. When the toxin is discovered and the person learns to avoid it, his/her health suddenly gets better.

For most people, though, the damage these toxic ingredients do is slow, and therefore very insidious. It can take decades to deteriorate your health to alarming levels. Since there are thousands of chemical culprits, finding out the ones that are creating the cellular malfunction can be like searching for a needle in the proverbial haystack.

That is why prevention is the solution, by giving your life a complete environmental makeover. Opt for natural and organic products and food in every area that is humanly possible. We recommend natural alternatives to toxic laundry products as a very good start in your quest for the proper functioning of the trillions of cells the comprise your body, so you will never be sick again.

In the past century, more than **80,000 known chemicals** have been introduced in our environment. The United States EPA (Environmental Protection Agency) only tests for about two hundred of them. Needless to say, the list of toxins that government agencies warn us to avoid is woefully inadequate, which is why you should avoid as many chemicals as possible.

One chemical that is not part of the 200 tested by the EPA is **1,4-dioxane**, a chemical known to **cause cancer, liver disease and other serious ailments**. It is found in many personal care products, including a number of detergents.

David Steinman from the Green Patriot Working Group (GPWG) began a study to see which consumer products are the worst offenders. This year, his organization along with the Organic Consumers Association (OCA), released the results of a portion of the study conducted last year on laundry detergents.

The top seven detergents with the highest concentration are:
Conventional brands:

1. Tide (P&G) – 55 parts per million (ppm)
2. Ivory Snow Gentle (P&G) – 31 ppm
3. Tide Free (P&G) – 29 ppm
4. Purex (Dial Corp.) – 25 ppm
5. Gain 2X Ultra (P&G) – 21 ppm
6. Cheer BrightClean Detergent (P&G) – 20 ppm
7. Era 2X Ultra (P&G) – 14 ppm
8. Arm & Hammer (Church & Dwight Co.) – 5.0 ppm
9. Wisk 2X Ultra (Sun Products Corp.) – 3.9 ppm
10. Woolite Complete Detergent (Reckitt Benckiser) – 1.3 ppm
11. All laundry detergent (Unilever) – 0.6 ppm
12. Dreft powdered detergent (P&G) – non-detectable (ND)
13. Sun Burst (Sun Products Corp.) – ND

"Natural" brands:

1. Planet Ultra Liquid laundry detergent– 6.1 ppm
2. Mrs. Meyers laundry detergent– 1.5 ppm
3. Clorox Green Works Natural laundry detergent – ND
4. Ecos laundry detergent (Earth Friendly Products) – ND
5. Life Tree Laundry Liquid– ND
6. Method Squeaky Green laundry detergent– ND
7. Seventh Generation Free & Clear laundry detergent – ND

Unfortunately, 1,4-dioxane is just the tip of the iceberg. To list all the harmful ingredients in laundry detergent, and all the studies indicating the potential health consequences of those chemicals, could easily fill a very large book. The solution is to change your lifestyle. Find natural alternatives to the chemicals you are using in your day to day life. They exist. You just have to look for them.

The Amazing Avocado

Beware of popular health myths. For instance, throughout the 1990s and into the first few years of this century, popular health "experts" often warned against eating coconut oil or coconut milk, causing many people to eschew a food now known to offer many health benefits. Another lingering popular health myth warns against avocados, which wrongly labels them as a dietary culprit because of their caloric and fat content. Yet, the truth is avocados can boost health in at least 5 ways:

1. Protein

Avocados provide all 18 essential amino acids necessary for the body to form a complete protein. Unlike the protein in steak, which is difficult for most people to digest, avocado protein is readily absorbed by the body because avocados also contain fiber. If you are trying to cut down on animal sources of protein in your diet, or if you are a vegetarian, vegan or raw foodist seeking more protein, avocados are a great nutritional ally to include not merely as an occasional treat, but as a regular part of your diet.

2. Beneficial Fats

Avocados provide the healthy kind of fat that your body needs. Like olive oil, avocadoes boost levels of HDL (the "good" cholesterol). HDL cholesterol can help protect against the damage caused by free radicals. This type of cholesterol also helps regulate triglyceride levels, preventing diabetes. A study published early this year in the *Canadian Medical Association Journal* found that a vegetarian diet, which includes HDL fats, can reduce levels of LDL (the "bad" cholesterol) as effectively as statin drugs.

3. Carotenoids

Avocados are an excellent source of carotenoids. Although many people associate carotenoids only with red and orange produce, avocadoes are also an excellent source of this phytonutrient. Avocadoes, also known as alligator pears, offer a diverse range of carotenoids including not only the better known ones such as beta-carotene, alpha-carotene and lutein, Every time you consume foods rich in carotenoids, you deliver high quality vitamin A to your body, thereby protecting eye health. Carotenoids also enhance the functioning of the immune system and promote healthy functioning of the reproductive system. Since carotenoids are fat soluble, eating avocados optimizes the absorption of these nutrients.

4. Anti-Inflammatory

The combined effect of the deluxe package of nutrients contained in avocados offers powerful anti-inflammatory benefits. Avocados' unique combination of Vitamins C and E, carotenoids, selenium, zinc, phytosterols and omega-3 fatty acids helps guard against inflammation. This means avocados can help prevent or mitigate against both osteo- and rheumatoid arthritis.

5. Heart Health

The fat content, which causes some uninformed health "experts" to deem avocados as unhealthy, actually provides protection against heart diseases. Studies have shown that oleic acid improves cardiovascular health. Oleic acid is the primary fatty acid in avocados. Many people now take supplements in order to consume more omega-3 fatty acids to lower their risk of heart disease. Avocados are rich in omega-3, delivering 160 milligrams per cup of alpha-linolenic acid.

Choosing and Eating

To get the most nutritional value from avocados, avoid those which have become over-ripe. You can identify these at the store because they will have dents and feel overly soft when you hold them. A ripe avocado should have no dents in its skin and will feel slightly soft when squeezed. You can also buy unripe avocados, which feel very hard when gripped, and permit them to ripen at home. The portion of the avocado closest to the skin is the densest in nutrients, so be sure to scrape the skin clean before discarding it.

Dangers of Birth Control

An easy and convenient method to prevent women from getting pregnant is through hormonal contraception or what we all know today as "the pill". It is a method of birth control in which a contraceptive is consumed by a female by mouth which can decrease the possibility of pregnancy for sexually active women if taken correctly and consistently. It can protect the female from unwanted pregnancy but it does not guard them against sexually transmitted diseases which include herpes and HIV virus. Today, an estimated 150 million women take oral contraceptives all around the world because of its easy accessibility. It is indeed true that some of these birth control pills can be bought over the counter and are readily available worldwide but the awareness of women for some of its health hazards have not been considered. Many women are not conscious of what these birth control pills do to their bodies which should have been a tantamount thing.

Firstly, understanding a woman's cycle is important in order to understand how birth control pills cause damage to the body. As a natural cycle, a woman's egg cell ripens every month and goes to the Fallopian tube for a period of time. A sperm can reach the egg there to be fertilized and journeys into the uterus to be implanted. The lining of the uterus gradually changes to accept the fertilized egg and prepare it for conception. But if the egg is not fertilized, the lining of the uterus sheds off, cleanse the reproductive system and continue the menstrual cycle for the following month.

How does a birth control pill work?

The natural cycle of the reproductive system is altered once birth control pills are taken because of the introduction of synthetic hormones. The synthetic progestin and estrogen in oral contraceptives disrupt the normal cycle of hormones to avoid pregnancy. Actually, there are combined factors to avoid the pregnancy. It can prevent the body to release a ripened egg from the ovary, alter the cervical plug to make the sperm immobile not reaching the egg before its viable period or change the cervical mucus lining to make it more difficult for a fertilized egg to be implanted. The abnormality of the reproductive cycle is what makes it hazardous to most women and yet it has been neglected by many. Aside from this disruption, emotional, psychological and mental aspects are also affected when contraceptives are taken. There are several pills that contains large amounts of synthetic hormones which greatly contributes to several side effects that women experience. Yet, only some of the doctors discuss the consequences of these pills.

Birth control pills change the physical aspect of a woman in response to the synthetic hormones introduced to the body. It can make the breasts larger and more tender, either increase or lessen the occurrence of acne, can contribute to **weight loss or gain**, **irregular bleeding and spotting**, and can make you feel nauseated or dizzy sometimes. It also affects your emotional state because of the fluctuating levels of hormones in your body. It can **create mood swings** before and after the menstrual cycle, can **intensify** your **depression** or may **lessen libido**.

A more serious health damage cause by birth control pills are the risks that accompany them. It **accelerates the risk of liver tumors** and cancers specifically **cervical and breast cancer**. It may lead to chest pains or heaviness which are important manifestations of a heart attack. It can also lead to speech impairment, numbness or weakness of an upper or lower extremity and a severe headache; all are definitive signs of having a stroke. Moreover, it can increase the existence of migraine. It can cause

gall bladder disease and infertility. Since birth control pills make the blood concentrated, it can contribute to:

- hypertension (high blood pressure)
- increased blood clotting that can lead to a vision loss when the blood clots in the eye area
- Irregular bleeding or spotting

In addition to this, there were also reported cases of liver damage and allergic reactions due to the intake of birth control pills. Liver manifestations include:

- dark urine
- upper right abdominal pain
- jaundice (yellow skin or eyes).

Signs of **allergic reactions** include itching, unexplained rashes or hives, unexplained swelling, wheezing and having a hard time swallowing or breathing.

Aside from diaphragms, cervical caps, condoms, and spermicides, there are many ways to **prevent pregnancy naturally** that are much safer for both men and women. If practiced correctly and in conjunction, the methods are highly effective and failure rates are very low.

8 of the World's Healthiest Spices & Herbs You Should Be Eating

Modern science is beginning to uncover the ultimate power of spices and herbs, as weapons against illnesses from cancer to Alzheimer's disease. "We're now starting to see a scientific basis for why people have been using spices medicinally for thousands of years.

In India, where spices tend to be used by the handful, incidence of diet-related diseases like heart disease and cancer have long been low. But when Indians move away and adopt more Westernized eating patterns, their rates of those diseases rise. While researchers usually blame the meatier, fattier nature of Western diets, many experts believe that herbs and spices-or more precisely, the lack of them-are also an important piece of the dietary puzzle. "When Indians eat more Westernized foods, they're getting much fewer spices than their traditional diet contains. "They lose the protection those spices are conveying."

While science has yet to show that any spice cures disease, there's compelling evidence that several may help manage some chronic conditions (though it's always smart to talk with your health care professional).

Chile Peppers May help: Boost metabolism. Chile peppers add a much-appreciated heat to chilly-weather dishes, and they can also give a boost to your metabolism. Thank capsaicin, the compound that gives fresh chilis, and spices including cayenne and chipotle, their kick. Studies show that capsaicin can increase the body's metabolic rate (causing one to burn more calories) and may stimulate brain chemicals that help us feel less hungry. In fact, one study found that people ate 16 percent fewer calories at a meal if they'd sipped a hot-pepper-spiked tomato juice (vs. plain tomato juice) half an hour earlier. Recent research found that capsinoids, similar but gentler chemicals found in milder chili hybrids, have the same effects-so even tamer sweet paprika packs a healthy punch. Capsaicin may also lower risk of ulcers by boosting the ability of stomach cells to resist infection by ulcer-causing bacteria and help the heart by keeping "bad" LDL cholesterol from turning into a more lethal, artery-clogging form.

Ginger May help: Soothe an upset stomach, fight arthritis pain. Ginger has a well-deserved reputation for relieving an unsettled stomach. Studies show ginger extracts can help reduce nausea caused by morning sickness or following surgery or chemotherapy, though it's less effective for motion sickness. But ginger is also packed with inflammation-fighting compounds, such as gingerols, which some experts believe may hold promise in fighting some cancers and may reduce the aches of osteoarthritis and soothe sore muscles. In a recent study, people who took ginger capsules daily for 11 days reported 25 percent less muscle pain when they performed exercises designed to strain their muscles (compared with a similar group taking placebo capsules). Another study found that ginger-extract injections helped relieve osteoarthritis pain of the knee.

Cinnamon May help: Stabilize blood sugar. A few studies suggest that adding cinnamon to food-up to a teaspoon a day, usually given in capsule form-might help people with type 2 diabetes better control their blood sugar, by lowering post-meal blood-sugar spikes. Other studies suggest the effects are limited at best.

Turmeric May help: Quell inflammation, inhibit tumors. Turmeric, the goldenrod-colored spice, is used in India to help wounds heal (it's applied as a paste); it's also made into a tea to relieve colds and respiratory problems. Modern medicine confirms some solid-gold health benefits as well; most are associated with curcumin, a compound in turmeric that has potent antioxidant and anti-inflammatory properties. Curcumin has been shown to help relieve pain of arthritis, injuries and dental procedures; it's also being studied for its potential in managing heart disease, diabetes and Alzheimer's disease. Researcher are bullish on curcumin's potential as a cancer treatment, particularly in colon, prostate and breast cancers; preliminary studies have found that curcumin can inhibit tumor cell growth and suppress enzymes that activate carcinogens.

Saffron May help: Lift your mood. Saffron has long been used in traditional Persian medicine as a mood lifter, usually steeped into a medicinal tea or used to prepare rice. Research from Iran's Roozbeh Psychiatric Hospital at Tehran University of Medical Sciences has found that saffron may help to relieve symptoms of premenstrual syndrome (PMS) and depression. In one study, 75% of women with PMS who were given saffron capsules daily reported that their PMS symptoms (such as mood swings and depression) declined by at least half, compared with only 8 percent of women who didn't take saffron.

Parsley May help: Inhibit breast cancer-cell growth. University of Missouri scientists found that this herb can actually inhibit breast cancer-cell growth, according to a study in September/October 2011 issue of EatingWell Magazine. In the study, animals that were given apigenin, a compound abundant in parsley (and in celery), boosted their resistance to developing cancerous tumors. Experts recommend adding a couple pinches of minced fresh parsley to your dishes daily.

Sage May help: Preserve memory, soothe sore throats. Herbalists recommend sipping sage tea for upset stomachs and sore throats, a remedy supported by one study that found spraying sore throats with a sage solution gave effective pain relief. And preliminary research suggests the herb may improve some symptoms of early Alzheimer's disease by preventing a key enzyme from destroying acetylcholine, a brain chemical involved in memory and learning. In another study, college students who took sage extracts in capsule form performed significantly better on memory tests, and their moods improved.

Rosemary May help: Enhance mental focus, fight foodborne bacteria. One recent study found that people performed better on memory and alertness tests when mists of aromatic rosemary oil were piped into their study cubicles. Rosemary is often used in marinades for meats and poultry, and there's scientific wisdom behind that tradition: rosmarinic acid and other antioxidant compounds in the herb fight bacteria and prevent meat from spoiling, and may even make cooked meats healthier. In March 2010, Kansas State University researchers reported that adding rosemary extracts to ground beef helped prevent the formation of heterocyclic amines (HCAs)-cancer-causing compounds produced when meats are grilled, broiled or fried.

How Long Can You Keep Foods?

Since I am not big juice drinker unless it's freshly squeezed, OJ usually only makes its way into my fridge when guests come to visit. I never thought much about keeping the OJ for a few weeks. After all, it still *tastes* good—and its usually finish before the expiration date. Then I read this study that showed opened OJ loses *all* antioxidant benefit after just one week! Seriously? Well, as you can imagine, this led me to wonder if other items in my kitchen lose their health punch over time.

Keep track of how long you store these items. Here's why: certain nutrients are unstable when exposed to oxygen (from the air), heat (from cooking) and light.

Orange juice: 1 week One cup of OJ can offer a full day's dose of vitamin C. But OJ that has been opened loses all antioxidant benefit after just one week. To get the most vitamin C, buy frozen concentrate and drink within a few days. Frozen concentrate is exposed to less light and air.

Green tea: 6 months A 2009 study in the *Journal of Food Science* showed that catechins (antioxidants linked with a reduced risk of some cancers) in green tea decreased markedly over time. After six months, catechin levels were 32 percent lower. Make the most of the antioxidants by storing tea in a sealed container in a dark, cool place.

Olive oil: 6 months Extra-virgin olive oil contains more than 45 heart-healthy antioxidants, but after six months of storage their potency decreases by about 40 percent, according to researchers at the University of Foggia in Italy. Why? Oxygen bubbles in the bottle destroy the antioxidants.

Honey: 6 months Researchers at the University of Illinois found the antioxidant power of clover and buckwheat honey decreased by 30 to 50 percent after six months. Consider buying buckwheat honey—it generally has more antioxidants to start with.

Knowledge of proper **food safety** is important in preventing food borne illness. If not refrigerated properly, foods become more susceptible to disease-causing bacteria. The US Department of Agriculture (USDA) recommends different amounts of time that food can be refrigerated, depending on the food group and whether it is fresh or processed. The USDA recommendations assume that refrigerator temperatures always remain at 40 F (or below). The amount of time that food is left out at room temperature should also be minimized. When food is left out at room temperature, bacteria starts to grow and the food begins to spoil. This article discusses different food groups and the amounts of time they can safety remain in the refrigerator.

Leftovers

Leftovers should not be left in the refrigerator longer than four days. If food has been left out for more than two hours, as a general rule, it should be discarded. When eating leftovers, the USDA advises reheating them to 325 degrees F. Reheating food to 325 degrees F or a higher temperature will eliminate bacteria. If leftovers are not consumed within 4 days, they should be stored in a freezer. If leftovers contain meat products, they should be eaten within two days of being refrigerated.

Dairy

When trying to determine if dairy has spoiled, you may think that you can just look for mold on cheese or curds in milk. Unfortunately, many molds begin growing before they are visible to the naked eye. This is why it is important to know how long dairy products should be kept in the fridge—this will keep you from defaulting to the "smell test" or looking for mold. If a milk carton is opened, the milk should be consumed within seven to ten days; even if that time is before the expiration date. Cheese varies depending on the variety. Harder cheeses stay fresh longer, with an average of three to four weeks, if opened. Soft cheese, like brie and ricotta, should be used within one week of opening.

Beef

Beef can be the source of many food borne illnesses. Common organisms such as staphylococcus, listeria, and E. coli are found in the intestines of cattle and can cause severe food borne illness if the beef is not refrigerated correctly. Different forms of beef have different protocols for refrigeration. Fresh beef and lunch meats should stay in the refrigerator no longer than three to five days after being opened. Canned beef can stay in the refrigerator three to four days after being opened. Homemade stews and dishes with beef cannot stay in the refrigerator longer than one to two days.

Chicken

Chicken contains many of the same bacteria as beef. Chicken also contains the bacterium campylobacter, which causes stomach upset. In order to reduce bacteria, fresh chicken can only safely stay in the refrigerator for one to two days. Cooked chicken such as rotisserie chicken, chicken nuggets and processed chicken can be refrigerated for three to four days. Chicken lunch meat can stay in the refrigerator for two weeks (if unopened); an opened package of chicken lunch meat will stay safe no longer than three to five days.

Health Benefits of Coconut Oil

The health benefits of **coconut oil** include hair care, skin care, stress relief, maintaining cholesterol levels, weight loss, increased immunity, proper digestion and metabolism, relief from kidney problems, heart diseases, high blood pressure, **diabetes**, HIV and **cancer**, dental care, and bone strength. These **benefits of coconut oil** can be attributed to the presence of lauric acid, capric acid and caprylic acid, and its properties such as antimicrobial, antioxidant, antifungal, antibacterial, soothing, etc.

How is Lauric Acid Used by our body?

The human body converts lauric acid into monolaurin which is claimed to help in dealing with viruses and bacteria causing diseases such as herpes, influenza, cytomegalovirus, and even **HIV**. It helps in fighting harmful bacteria such as listeria monocytogenes and helicobacter pylori, and harmful protozoa such as giardia lamblia. As a result of these various health benefits of coconut oil, though its exact mechanism of action was unknown, it has been extensively used in Ayurveda, the traditional Indian medicinal system. **The Coconut Research Center** has compiled various references on **scientific research done on coconut oil**.

Before we move on to the benefits of coconut oil in detail, let us understand its composition.

Composition of Coconut Oil:

- Coconut oil consists of more than ninety percent of saturated fats (Don't panic! First read to the last word. Your opinion may change), with traces of few unsaturated fatty acids, such as monounsaturated fatty acids and polyunsaturated fatty acids. **Virgin Coconut Oil** is no different from this.

Let us now explore the benefits of coconut oil in detail:

Hair Care:

Coconut oil is one of the best natural nutrition for hair. It helps in healthy growth of hair providing them a shiny complexion. Regular **massage** of the head with coconut oil ensures that your scalp is free of dandruff, lice, and lice eggs, even if your scalp is dry. Coconut oil is extensively used in the Indian sub-continent for hair care. It is an excellent conditioner and helps in the re-growth of damaged hair. It also provides the essential proteins required for nourishing damaged hair. It is therefore used as hair care oil and used in manufacturing various conditioners, and dandruff relief creams. Coconut oil is normally applied topically for **hair care**.

Skin Care:

Coconut oil is excellent **massage oil** for the skin as well. It acts as an effective moisturizer on all types of skins including **dry skin**. The benefit of coconut oil on the skin is comparable to that of mineral oil. Further, unlike mineral oil, there is no chance of having any adverse side effects on the skin with the application of coconut oil. Coconut oil therefore is a safe solution for preventing dryness and flaking of skin. It also delays wrinkles, and sagging of skin which normally become prominent with age. Coconut oil also helps in treating various skin problems including psoriasis, dermatitis, **eczema** and other **skin infections**. Therefore, coconut oil forms the basic ingredient of various **body care** products such as soaps, lotions, creams, etc., used for skin care. Coconut oil also helps in preventing **premature aging** and degenerative diseases due to its antioxidant properties.

Heart Diseases:

There is a misconception spread among many people that coconut oil is not good for the heart. This is because it contains a large quantity of saturated fats. However, coconut oil is beneficial for the heart. It contains about 50% lauric acid, which helps in preventing various heart problems including high cholesterol levels and high blood pressure.

The saturated fats present in coconut oil are not harmful as it happens in case of other **vegetables** oils. It does not lead to increase in LDL levels. It also reduces the incidence of injury in arteries and therefore helps in preventing atherosclerosis.

Weight Loss

Coconut oil is very useful in **reducing weight**. It contains short and medium-chain fatty acids that help in taking off excessive weight. It is also easy to digest and it helps in healthy functioning of the thyroid and enzymes systems. Further, it increases the body metabolism by removing stress on pancreases, thereby burning out more energy and helping obese and overweight people reduce their weight. Hence, people living in tropical coastal areas, who eat coconut oil daily as their primary cooking oil, are normally not fat, obese or overweight.

Digestion

Internal use of coconut oil occurs primarily as cooking oil. Coconut oil helps in improving the digestive system and thus prevents various stomach and digestion related problems including irritable bowel syndrome. The saturated fats present in coconut oil have anti -microbial properties and help in dealing with various bacteria, fungi, parasites, etc., that cause indigestion. Coconut oil also helps in absorption of other nutrients such as vitamins, **minerals** and amino acids.

Immunity:

Coconut oil is also good for the immune system. It strengthens the immune system as it contains antimicrobial lipids, lauric acid, capric acid and caprylic acid which have antifungal, antibacterial and antiviral properties. The human body converts lauric acid into monolaurin which is claimed to help in dealing with viruses and bacteria causing diseases such as herpes, influenza, cytomegalovirus, and even **HIV**. It helps in fighting harmful bacteria such as listeria monocytogenes and helicobacter pylori.

Healing and Infections

When applied on infections, it forms a chemical layer which protects the infected body part from external **dust**, air, fungi, bacteria and virus. Coconut oil is most effective on **bruises** as it speeds up the healing process by repairing damaged tissues.

Infections: Coconut oil is very effective against a variety of infections due to its antifungal, antiviral, and antibacterial properties. According to the **Coconut Research Center**, coconut oil kills viruses that cause influenza, measles, hepatitis, herpes, SARS, etc. It also kills bacteria that cause ulcers, throat infections, urinary tract infections, pneumonia, and gonorrhea, etc. Coconut oil is also effective on fungi and yeast that cause candida, ringworm, **athlete's foot**, **diaper rash**, etc.

Is Collagen Type II A Cure for Arthritis and Heart Disease?

According to the latest statistics, 50 million Americans suffer from some form of arthritis, either rheumatoid or osteoarthritis, as well as a variety of other arthritic conditions. All forms of arthritis share the common symptoms of severe pain, loss of range of motion, and a diminished quality of life. Add to this the fact that the number one killer in our country today is still cardiovascular disease, and you have all of the conditions necessary for a plethora of pharmaceutical and natural medicines designed to reduce the severity of these diseases. Could it be that one nutritional medicine called collagen type II can cure both disorders in an effective way? Safety also becomes an issue. Currently modern medicines, such as nonsteroidal anti-inflammatories (NSAIDS), can cause occult bleeding, ulcers and even life-threatening side effects. Other approaches include natural medicines such as fish liver oil, and shark cartilage. It may turn out that the natural components of cartilage hold the greatest promise of helping both arthritis and heart disease.

We know that cartilage is composed of four or five different kinds of collagen. There are 14 different kinds of collagen altogether, but the primary collagen, the most predominant one, the most medicinal collagen, is collagen type II. If collagen type II is derived from chicken sternal cartilage, from chicks six to eight weeks old, it contains the greatest number of anti-inflammatory and joint supporting agents.

These agents include glucosamine sulfate which has over 30 years of double-blind, placebo-controlled studies indicating that it actually helps to rebuild the cartilage in arthritis joints. We also know that it contains a high concentration of chondroitin sulfate A, which is a powerful anti-inflammatory and also supports the joint tissue. Once again, if the product is derived from chicken sternal cartilage, these two components are in highest concentration compared to any other cartilage source. In addition to these, collagen type II also contains a powerful, newly discovered antioxidant agent called cartilage matrix glycoprotein (CMGP), which can help reduce the oxidative damage to the joint. In addition to these new discoveries, there are other ingredients in collagen type II that make it more effective than just taking glucosamine or chondroitin by themselves. Another advantage of collagen type II over cartilage is that it is much more absorbable, Researchers have recently demonstrated about eight percent absorption of ground cartilage, whereas the components of collagen type II have a much higher absorption rate of 70 to 90 percent. This means considerably less collagen type II has to be taken in comparison to cartilage. Most people have to take 9 to 12 grams of cartilage in order to get a response, whereas with collagen type II as little as two grams, and more commonly three to four grams, are quite sufficient. When people suffer from arthritis, there is a selective destruction of collagen type II in the joint cartilage itself. Scientists know that this particular component of cartilage is being attacked by white blood cells and somehow this activates the immune system in the rheumatoid arthritis patient to develop antibodies to collagen type II. This then sets up an immune response to all of the cartilage that is degenerating in the body. Thus, both wrists hurt, both knees hurt, the hips, the back, etc. In osteoarthritis, we have a wear and tear type of destruction of the cartilage with the release of soluble collagen type II, but without the immune response. The end result is the same. Pain, more pain, and loss of quality of life. The question now becomes how does collagen type II turn off the immune system in the rheumatoid arthritis. The answer is that collagen type II's effectiveness is accomplished through "oral tolerance."

Collagen type II also contains agents that inhibit blood vessel formation in joints and reduce enzyme attacks on the cartilage itself. Thus, there is a rejuvenation of the cartilage producing cells and a decrease in the destructive biochemistry of the joint. Additionally, many of these agents found in collagen type II support the lubricating fluid of the joint called the synovial fluid. These agents increase the thickness and lubricating effectiveness of this fluid. It is extremely important to understand that not all types of collagen are the same, and not all types of cartilage can give you a medicinally effective collagen type II. Collagen type II must be derived from chicken sternal cartilage, only. The reason is very simple. This source of cartilage holds the greatest concentration of joint-saving proteoglycans. When a person who has arthritis begins to take collagen type II, they should wait of a period of four to eight weeks before they decide as to whether or not the product is working. It takes this length of time in most people to get significant results. We have heard some individuals eliminate pain within one week, but this is the exception, not the rule. Collagen type II is available in 500 mg. capsules. It should be taken in divided doses throughout the day - 20 minutes before eating, preferably with a small amount of orange juice as this improves absorption. In lieu of the fact that there are no side effects with collagen type II, this would seem to be the product of choice when suffering from any form of arthritic condition. https://www.npscript.com/dougcaporrino/joint-revitalizer/VI0065PAR

The Miracle of Wheatgrass

What's in Wheatgrass Juice?
Why should I drink wheatgrass juice?

Wheatgrass juice will provide you with more energy by fulfilling nutritional deficiencies and by removing wastes that clog your cells, blood, tissues and organs. I firmly believe that even so called "healthy" people can live their lives at an even higher level of energy and mental concentration. We have all read the horror stories concerning environmental hazards that our bodies are subjected to as a result of our highly developed industrial and technical lifestyles: all forms of pollution (air, water, sound, etc.); chemicals in our food and water; radiation given out by televisions, computers, and other high-tech machines; and so on. When the body is subjected to these hazards it loses its balance, resulting in loss of energy, inability to concentrate, and depression, not to mention other more devastating degenerative conditions. It has been scientifically shown that wheatgrass juice neutralizes these environmental toxins, allowing the body to balance itself and operate at maximum efficiency.

How much wheatgrass juice should I drink each day?

As a daily nutritional supplement and "environmental- hazard neutralizer", I would recommend 1 or 2 ounces per day, taken on an empty stomach, preferably before a meal. If a juicer is un available, the grass can be chewed and the pulp discarded. Take a little in your mouth at a time and let it sit there for 30 to 45 seconds before swallowing, this will aid in the digestion of it.

Wheatgrass, is not a supplement. It is a complete food.

Of all the valuable compounds contained in wheatgrass juice, chlorophyll is one of the most important. If it were not for its delicate nature, I think it would be one of the top weapons in the medical arsenal. Its instability is of no concern to us, however, because we can grow, juice, and drink wheatgrass without having to store it for long periods.

What is chlorophyll?

Chlorophyll is a proteinous compound found in the green leaves of plants and grasses. It converts the sun's energy into a form that plants, animals and people can use. Thus, it is sort of a living battery. Also important is its remarkable similarity to hemoglobin, the compound that carries oxygen in the blood. We have all read that an oxygen-rich body is a healthy one.

The nutritional structure of wheatgrass is very close to that of our body; in other words, it contains all of the necessary vitamins, minerals and protein that our body needs. I do want to say, now, that wheatgrass juice provides these elements together in exact proportions that nature intended. NO SUPPLEMENTS with their quantities can provide the body with the nutrients found in wheatgrass juice.

Nutritionally, wheatgrass contains about the same amount of Vitamin C as citrus and other fruits, and more than common vegetables like tomatoes or potatoes. As you know, Vitamin C is important to the health of the skin, teeth, gums, muscles, and joints. It also aids general growth and development and acts as an antioxidant.

Wheatgrass juice supplies about as much Vitamin A as dark green varieties of lettuce and more than most fruits. Vitamin A is essential for normal growth and development, good eyesight, and reproduction. The Vitamin A found in liver, fish oils, animal foods, and most vitamin supplements accumulates in the liver and can become toxic in large doses.

Vitamin E is a fat-soluble vitamin, without enough of it we would face muscle degeneration, sterility, and slower healing of wounds and infections. Vitamin E, an antioxidant and fertility vitamin, is also a protector of the heart. The type of Vitamin E found in wheatgrass is about ten times more easily assimilated by the body than any of the synthetic varieties. Wheatgrass is a good source of calcium, which helps build strong bones and teeth and regulates heartbeat, in addition to acting as a buffer to restore balance to blood pH.

Keep in mind calcium cannot be properly absorbed unless other trace minerals are present along with it. Wheatgrass, as I said before, contains the optimal balance of vitamins and minerals so that all nutrients, especially calcium, are properly absorbed.

Our bodies do need sodium to aid digestion and elimination, and to regulate the amount of fluid in the body. However, most Americans consume far too much it in the form of sodium chloride and in food additives such as MSG. One proof of our need for sodium is the fact that our normal blood contains five (5 gr.!) grams per pint. Wow! Wheatgrass, as expected, provides *only* this minute amount, thus making it an ideal and safe for those on a sodium-restricted diet.

Without enough iron, we can easily become tired or anemic as many women's health do during menstruation due to loss of iron. Inorganic iron is often constipating, but the iron salts in wheatgrass have no side effects. In juice form, wheatgrass contains about half as much iron as spinach or other greens that are good sources of iron. Unlike spinach, beet greens, or chard, however, wheatgrass contains little or no oxalic acid — an element in the foods I just mentioned that binds the useable calcium in the system and can leach calcium from teeth and bones, and cause kidney stones.

Potassium, called the youth mineral by some nutritionists, helps maintain a smooth mineral balance, and balanced body weight. It also tones the muscles, firms the skin, and promotes overall beauty. (So, does MSM.) Fruits, especially bananas, are well-known for their good supply of potassium. Wheatgrass juice contains about as much potassium as citrus fruits, grapes, apples and melons.

You will find about as much magnesium in wheatgrass as in broccoli, Brussel sprouts, beets, carrots, or celery. Magnesium is important for good muscle function and for bowel health, as it aids eliminative functions. I believe that this mineral is also responsible for drawing fat out of the liver, in cases of fatty infiltration there.

More than 50 percent of the dry weight of our body is protein. We therefore need to eat foods that contain a protein structure nearly identical to our body's. The protein found in meat and dairy is far from having the ideal protein structure. This structure is further distorted by cooking. A meat- and dairy-eating body overworks to adapt to these foreign protein sources, and learns how to extract and reform necessary nutrients. the unused portions, wastes, are then stored in the body as fat and other toxic residues. When the work becomes overwhelming for the body, it begins to degenerate, causing a breakdown of the immune system and structural damage to organs and body tissue. It makes much more sense to ingest protein that resembles the protein structure in our body. Wheatgrass juice protein is the optimal form of protein.

Proteins are composed of smaller proteinous "chains" called amino acids. Amino acids can be compared with raw materials used in building a house, whereas enzymes do the actual building. Together, enzymes and amino acids are responsible for cell renewal and a huge array of diverse functions, from the creation of hormones to the building up of muscles, blood, and organs.

Again, I want to stress that we cannot separate the body elements as they do in the laboratory. All amino acids are necessary in the proper proportions, as found in wheatgrass juice. When we separate these and try to take large doses of any particular element, we create a body imbalance.

Amino acids are involved in many systems and functions. Let's just say that they are essential to proper digestion and assimilation of foods, strong immunity from disease, rapid healing of cuts and wounds, proper liver function, and regulation of our mental awareness. Above all, the action of the amino acids on cells in the process of self-renewal rejuvenates us and prolongs life. A deficiency of just one amino acid can easily result in allergies, low energy, sluggish digestion, poor resistance to infection, and premature aging. The replacement of that amino acid can easily result in the complete reversal of these symptoms. In essence, adequate supply of amino acids is the difference between fair health and low energy levels, and, mental clarity, and strong resistance to germs and other microbes.

Lysine is one amino acid that is receiving attention as a potential anti-aging factor. Body growth and blood circulation are fostered by this important amino acid. Without enough lysine, our immune response weakens, sight may be affected, and fatigue occur. Another essential, isoleucine, is also needed for growth, especially in infants, and for protein balance in adults. A deficiency of isoleucine could end in mental retardation, as it affects the production of other amino acids.

Leucine is an amino acid that keeps us alert and awake. An adequate supply of leucine is necessary for anyone who wants to experience high-energy living.

Another amino acid you may have heard of is tryptophan. It is essential for building rich, red blood, healthy skin, and hair. Working with the B-complex vitamins, tryptophan also helps to calm nerves and stimulate better digestion.

One of the other great 8 eight essential amino acids in methionine, which helps cleanse and regenerate kidney and liver cells. It also may stimulate hair growth and mental calmness. Its effect is nearly opposite that of leucine; methionine calms rather than hypes the emotions and mental processes.

Briefly, some of the other amino acids in wheatgrass are: alanine, a blood purifier; arginine, which is especially vital to men's health, aspartic acid, a helper in the conversion of food into energy; glutamic acid, which improves mental balance and provides for smooth metabolic function; glycine, a helper in the process whereby cells use oxygen to make energy; histidine, which seems to affect hearing and nervous functions; proline, which becomes glutamic acid and performs the same tasks; serine, a stimulator of the brain and nerve functions; tyrosine, which aids the formation of hair and skin and prevents cellular aging.

In essence, the same life force in nature that explodes into groceries every spring can be transferred into the human body via the consumption of wheatgrass juice. The body can then use this super-nutritious, vital energy to heal and grow young.

Don't Take These Pain Killers

We all hope it will never happen. But if it does, you might be surprised to discover that when it comes to fracture healing, the "don'ts" may be just as important as the "do's".

I'm talking about the recent discovery that pain killers inhibit the body's ability to heal fractures. This includes COX-2 inhibitor drugs such as Celebrex and other commonly used non-steroidal anti-inflammatory drugs (NSAIDs) such as Aleve, Motrin and aspirin.

Let's face it, a broken bone hurts a whole lot, so it is not surprising that it has become almost an instinct to reach out for the drugs. But the consequences of this can mean a much longer recovery period.

How do These Drugs Work?

NSAIDs are mostly COX-1 and slightly COX-2 inhibitors. These are fatty-acid derivatives located all over the body that react to immune and inflammatory conditions. COX-1 also protect the stomach by producing mucus and increasing the production of sodium bicarbonate, maintain blood flow and kidney function, and process sensations.

So, COX-2 inhibitors were developed as a more targeted prescription drug that would spare the stomach lining from damage. In fact, drugs like Celebrex (celecoxib) and the infamous Vioxx and Bextra entered the market as a 'safer' NSAID replacement, but with disastrous results. You might recall that Vioxx was voluntarily withdrawn from the market in

September 2004 by Merck, its manufacturer. Less than one year later, Bextra was black-listed as well.

The How to of Fracture Healing

There are four phases in fracture healing. Immediately after a bone breaks, the body starts the healing process. Next, there is tremendous inflammation followed by a regenerative phase characterized by new bone growth. The last phase involves remodeling, in which mature bone is replaced by newly formed bone.

The early inflammation serves a very important purpose, since the chemical signals released during this phase are critical in sustaining the healing process. So, it makes sense that anti-inflammatory drugs alter the messaging system and wreak havoc in the fracture healing process.

Science Proves Yet Again That Nature Knows Best

A study conducted on laboratory rats and published in the Journal of Joint and Bone Surgery used COX-2 inhibitors to gage the dosage and subsequent healing delay of thigh bone fractures.1 Interestingly, fracture healing inhibition was evident regardless of the COX-2 dose. But the most noticeable healing delay happened with treatment lasting longer than 15 days.

The researchers concluded that the same can be said about "regular" NSAIDs and recommend avoiding NSAIDs after a fracture.

This is one more proof that Nature knows best. Because even though pain can be very unpleasant, rushing to intervene and stop the inflammation following injury disrupts the inflammatory response. There is a good reason for all that swelling, heat, and redness; it is a sign of increased blood flow to the area. And increased blood flow means the body can clear debris away from the site of injury and begin with the healing process.2

Most Popular NSAIDs

Here are the over-the-counter and prescription NSAIDs most commonly used:

- Aspirin (Bayer, Bufferin)
- Ibuprofen (Motrin, Advil)

- Ketoprofen (Orudis)
- Piroxicam (Feldene)
- Naproxen (Aleve, Naprosyn)
- Indomethacin (Indocin)
- Daypro
- Celebrex

Try This Colorful Cure

So, what to do for pain, you might rightly ask? There are many ways to naturally deal with it. Here's one that works and is chock-full of nutrients: beets. Studies have shown that beets inhibit COX-1 and COX-2, thanks to their rich content of betanin, and isobetanin, the specific phytonutrients responsible for their anti-inflammatory action. Beet juice as well as beet root juice is loaded with COX-1 & COX-2 inhibitors. You can juice several times a week using organic beets only.

What Color is Your Poop?

When your body's gastrointestinal tract isn't functioning correctly, stool colors can tell you what's going on in your insides and whether you might have bowel problems.

The color of stool normally is brown. The reason for the brown color is the presence of bile in the stool. Bile is made by the liver, concentrated and stored in the gallbladder, and secreted into the intestine to aid in the digestion of food. Depending on the amount of bile it contains, the normal stool color can range in color from light yellow to almost black.

Bile secreted from the gallbladder into the intestine is a very dark green liquid made up of many chemicals, one of which is bilirubin. When red blood cells are destroyed naturally in the body, the hemoglobin, a protein inside the red blood cells that carries oxygen, is modified in the liver. The by-product of this process is bilirubin, and the liver secretes the bilirubin into bile.

As the bile travels through the intestines, it can undergo further chemical changes, and its color can also change. For example, if the traveling time through the intestine is too rapid, then bile won't have the time to go through additional color changes and the stool color may be close to green.

The color of stool can change for other reasons as well. Many changes in stool color may not be of much importance, especially if the change happens once and is not consistent from one stool to the next. Sudden major changes in stool color that persist may suggest an underlying medical problem. Furthermore, gradual but persistent changes in stool color also can signify medical problems.

Medium brown is the color of healthy poop.

Pale, gray, clay-like stool suggests a liver problem. Bile from the liver is what makes stools brown; not enough and you get ashy shades indicating anything from gallstones to hepatitis, pancreatitis to cirrhosis.

Black or dull red stool sounds scary, but is often related to food or meds. You may see black after consuming black licorice, blueberries, iron pills, or Pepto-Bismol. (Call your doc if you see *tarry* black poop, which can be a sign of bleeding in the upper intestines or even the stomach.) And red? That may come from beets and tomatoes.

Green stools aren't just for St. Patrick's Day, although they can be from celebratory beer (it's the green dye). Greenies can also come from eating lots of green vegetables or taking iron or certain medications.

Bloody or maroon/red poop is most often caused by hemorrhoids but it can also be from intestinal bleeding, so call your doc.

The Truth About Cereal

We live in a time where processed and genetically modified (GM/GMO) foods have become normal and are creeping into our kitchens. However, will you be alright buying your usual breakfast cereal knowing some of the things that are in it? Far from being a scare tactic, this statement is the outcome of the several news reports, studies, and undercover investigations that have revealed a majority of 'fortified', 'organic', and 'nutritious' cereals may not always live up to their claims.

The pressing concern is the fact that many well reputed and established multinational corporations (MNCs) are guilty of misleading consumers and even putting their lives at stake. Here's a compilation of some of the most indicting headlines and findings over the last few years about the once-revered all American staple- cereal.

Kellogg's in the rut

In 2004, one of America's (and the world's) most well-known food brands, Kellogg's, was made to eat humble pie when it was forced to recall its line of cereals that had come packaged with the 'Spidey Signal' toy.

Shockingly, these toys consisted of mercury batteries, which meant that there was a serious risk of the cereal being contaminated due to probable exposure to the batteries. Apart from the risk of food contamination or poisoning, there was also a hue and cry over the environmental pollution aspect, since the toys were easily disposable. This increased the likelihood of certain safety standards pertaining to waste disposal being violated or not adhered to.

As a result, the Spidey Signal toy was withdrawn from the market in states like Connecticut, New York, and New Hampshire.

However, that wasn't all. In the same year, Denmark declared a ban on the addition of folic acid, calcium, iron, and vitamins and minerals in all Kellogg's products. This step was taken because the Danish government established that such food products contained 'toxic doses' of all the above and could endanger the lives of pregnant women and young children.

Deadly toxins in a box

In March 2011, news broke out about research studies and tests in Switzerland and Germany that were conducted on cardboard boxes widely used as packaging for foods like cereal, bread, pasta, rice, etc. The results of these laboratory tests were shocking.

It was revealed that an overwhelming majority of these boxes contained dangerously high levels- up to 100 times the permissible limit- of chemicals like mineral oil hydrocarbon.

Mineral oil hydrocarbons are detrimental to the organs and also increase cancer risk in individuals.

After the findings became public, popular cereal makers like Weetabix, Kellogg's, and Jordan's, an English brand, were forced to reconsider their packaging practices. However, what made the results of this study even more derogatory was the fact that in 2010, Kellogg's in the USA had been forced to withdraw 28 million cereal boxes from the market after consumers across the nation complained of foul smells, leached chemicals seeping through the boxes, and queasiness.

Of the 119 products that were tested during this study, only 30 products were deemed chemical and toxin free as they had a better inner barrier lining. Most of the foods that 'failed' in this test had recycled paper wrapping which contained traces of newspaper ink.

In August of 2018 renowned Toxicologist Alexis Temkin, Ph.D., Toxicologist wrote a story uncovering the toxic effects of Glyphosate in children's cereals.

Popular oat cereals, oatmeal, granola and snack bars come with a hefty dose of the weed-killing poison in Roundup, according to independent laboratory tests commissioned by EWG.

Glyphosate, an herbicide linked to cancer by California state scientists and the World Health Organization, was found in all but two of 45 samples of products made with conventionally grown oats. Almost three-fourths of those samples had glyphosate levels higher than what EWG scientists consider protective of children's health with an adequate margin of safety. About one-third of 16 samples made with organically grown oats also had glyphosate, all at levels well below EWG's health benchmark.

Glyphosate is the active ingredient in Roundup, the Monsanto weed killer that is the most heavily used pesticide in the U.S. Last week, a California jury ordered Monsanto to pay $289 million in damages to a man dying of cancer, which he says was caused by his repeated exposure to large quantities of Roundup and other glyphosate-based weed killers while working as a school groundskeeper.

EWG tested more than a dozen brands of oat-based foods to give Americans information about dietary exposures that government regulators are keeping secret. In April, internal emails obtained by the nonprofit US Right to Know revealed that the Food and Drug Administration has been testing food for glyphosate for two years and has found "a fair amount," but the FDA has not released its findings.

'Natural'? Not really

How many times have you walked down the aisle in a grocery store or supermarket and had hundreds of 'organic', 'natural', or 'fortified' cereal boxes staring at you from the shelves? Chances are that you may have purchased such products several times over after believing they live up to their promises.

The truth, however, is a different matter altogether.

Deceptive labeling and advertising practices are adopted by too many cereal manufacturers, due to which consumers are easily cheated and misled into thinking what they are buying is genuinely good for them when it isn't. An undercover investigation by Cornucopia Institute to determine whether so-called organic/natural cereals are indeed what they claim to be was carried out in 2011, after which the organization published the results via a 'cereal scorecard' on its site. The parameters were: whether the cereal was genetically modified, contained toxic chemicals and/or pesticides, or consisted of other 'non-natural' elements.

Cornucopia Institute's scorecard proved that most cereal brands which claimed some of their products were either organic or natural were deceiving customers. A majority of the samples proved that most 'natural' breakfast cereals by General Mills, Kashi, Mom's Best, Barbara's Bakery, Whole Foods, Health Valley, *et al* were, in fact, either manufactured with genetically modified (GM) corn, soy, grains, etc., or contained synthetic/chemical ingredients.

Conclusion

True natural and/or organic cereal seems to have become a rarity, but you can take heart in the fact that there are a few genuine cereal brands out there that have a stellar reputation for living up to all their claims. These include the likes of Nature's Path, Country Choice Organic, Ambrosial, Go Raw, and many more that have been listed on the Cornucopia Institute website.

If you are inclined, you can also make your own cereal at home. There are innumerable recipe websites that outline the many ways in which you can creatively concoct your own granola and cereal with only the choicest, most wholesome ingredients.

Green Tea Prevents Kidney Stones

According to traditional medical wisdom, if you want to avoid kidney problems, you'd better avoid tea. Tea has high oxalate content, and since the most common type of kidney stone builds on oxalic acid, drinking tea is verboten for kidney stone patients. But recent research suggests, though it seems counterintuitive, that green tea actually helps minimize the risk of kidney stones.

About five percent of people worldwide get kidney stones, and those people do suffer. Kidney stones can be extremely painful. They occur when crystalline masses form in the urine, and in 80 percent of stones, those crystals are based on oxalate combined with calcium. If large enough, the stones can create agonizing obstructions in the urinary tract and block the flow of urine out of the kidneys. Symptoms, in addition to plain old agony, can include swelling of the kidneys, nausea, vomiting, blood in the urine, and fever. Fortunately, the urine normally contains a substance that breaks down the stones, and so most stones remain small and just pass out of the body without major event.

But some people lack enough of the dissolving factor in their urine, plus, certain types of food interfere with the normal process of dissolving stones or actually add to the stones. Tops on the list are foods high in oxalic acid, such as spinach, beans, tofu, chocolate, wheat brain, nuts, strawberries, coffee — and tea. In fact, coffee and tea typically top the list of dietary restrictions for the stone sensitive, so the discovery that green tea may actually prevent stones comes as a surprise. It seems that green tea binds to calcium oxalate, creating flat crystals that break down more easily than other shapes. The more green tea the stones are exposed to, the flatter the stones become.

The research team that discovered the phenomenon comes from Sichuan University in, China. They grew calcium oxalate crystals and then studied the effect of exposing the crystals to various conditions and substances. Their results suggest that drinking green tea might be a good habit for the prevention of human stone formation,"

Previous studies also noted the beneficial action of green tea on kidney stones, but researchers couldn't make sense of the finding, and so tea held its place on the forbidden list for kidney stone victims. A study published in the *Annals of Internal Medicine* in 1998 reported on a study of 81,093 women aged 40 to 86 years of with no history of kidney stones. The study found that for each cup of green tea consumed daily, the subjects reduced the risk of kidney stones by eight percent. A parallel study found that for each cup of tea that men drank, their risk of kidney stones went down by a whopping 14 percent! Again, these findings confounded scientists, since the levels of calcium oxalate in urine increased as subjects increased their intake of tea, and as stated earlier, high levels of oxalates usually mean more vulnerability to kidney stones. But this latest research finally sheds light on the green tea factor. Oxalate level isn't everything — it's how it affects the crystals that counts.

Also, it's noteworthy that teas vary considerably in their oxalate content. While black tea contains between about 4.6 and 5.1 milligrams per gram, green tea contains only a fraction of that amount —.23 to 1.15 milligrams per gram. The huge difference in oxalate content would at worst render green tea less harmful than black tea, even without its propensity to bind to calcium oxalate. And at best, by drinking green tea, you prevent kidney stones while reaping the benefits of the high catechin content — including inhibiting tumor growth, regulating blood sugar, reducing cholesterol and triglycerides, and reversing the ravages of heart disease.

As for the kidney stones, it's best to prevent them in the first place. You minimize the chances of getting stones if you drink enough water, avoid sodas and sports drinks, minimize salt intake, eat a balanced diet rich in vegetables and fruits, and refrain from overloading on oxalate-rich foods. And, of course, when it comes to kidney stones, nothing works faster or is more effective than a well-designed herbal kidney flush formula. A good formula can start providing benefits in as little as one hour.

A Kidney Care Formula

As the incidence of kidney problems has soared to epidemic levels over the last ten years, the need for a strong, dedicated formula for doing a regular kidney detox has become paramount. Even though a number of herbs (chanca piedra, juniper berry, uva ursi, parsley root, dandelion root, and horsetail) are common to both kidney and liver maintenance, a few additional ingredients are necessary for long-term kidney health. Such a kidney detox formula should also play a major role in eliminating gallstones and, amazingly, even helping with arthritis.

But first, let's explore some background on the kidneys and the extent of the problem in the world today.

The Kidneys

The kidneys are bean-shaped organs located on either side of the lower back, just below the rib cage. Their function is to:

- Keep the composition of your blood balanced.
- Regulate the amount of fluid in the body.
- Control balance of electrolytes in your blood.
- Help to control blood pressure.
- Produce hormones that are crucial for blood and bone formation.

After blood is filtered through the kidneys, the primary byproduct is urine. The production of urine is a complex process. Far from being a simple removal of water from the body, it is, rather, a process of selective filtration that not only removes waste and potential toxins from the blood while retaining essential molecules, but that also serves to balance key biochemicals and hormones in the blood. Blood enters the kidneys by way of the renal artery and is processed in tiny tubes called nephrons and returned to circulation through the renal veins. The substances that are filtered are turned into urine, composed of 95% water, 2.5% urea, 2.5% mixture of minerals, salt, hormones and enzymes. Urine is then collected in the central part of the kidney and passes through the ureters to the bladder. When the bladder is full of urine, it is emptied from the body through the urethra. Approximately 180 liters of blood move through the two kidneys every day, about 1.5 liters of urine are produced.

Other Functions of the Kidneys

In addition to cleaning the blood, the kidneys regulate the amount of water contained in the blood. ADH (Vasopressin) is an anti-diuretic hormone produced in the hypothalamus and stored in the pituitary gland. When the amount of salt and other substances in the blood becomes too high, the pituitary glands release ADH into the bloodstream and to the kidneys. This increases the permeability of the walls of the renal tubules, helping to reabsorb more water into the blood stream. **The kidneys also adjust the body's acid-base balance to prevent acidosis and alkalosis.**

Another function of the kidneys is the processing of vitamin D. The kidneys convert this vitamin to an active form that stimulates bone development.

The nephrons

As mentioned above, the processing (or filtering) in the kidneys is done in the nephrons. Not surprisingly then, most kidney problems are focused in the nephrons, and correspondingly, most kidney drugs target the nephrons. For example, most diuretics inhibit the ability of the nephrons to retain water, thereby increasing the amount of urine produced.

The important thing to understand about the nephrons is that they are very, very tiny – and therefore easily plugged. When plugged, they become inflamed and infected and die. Also, because they are so small they are easily damaged by chemical imbalances in the blood that attack protein – specifically, high blood sugar and high insulin – which is why diabetes and kidney disease go hand in hand. The bottom line is that over time, when enough nephrons die, kidney function is compromised to the point that the kidneys can no longer do their job. At that point they require outside support (i.e. dialysis) or outright replacement (a kidney transplant).

Kidney Diseases

Diseases of the kidneys range from mild infection to life-threatening kidney failure. The most common form of kidney disease is an inflammation of the kidneys. Kidney sludge is the result of the accumulated crystallized minerals that sometimes obstruct the flow of urine and damage the kidneys. If the minerals accumulate to a sufficient degree, the sludge actually forms into rough surfaced stones that actually rip and tear at the ureters on their way out of the kidneys.

Anyone who suffers from kidney stones knows the pain involved in passing a stone, but keep in mind that a kidney stone is only the extreme manifestation of sludge. Just because you don't suffer from kidney stones doesn't mean you don't have a problem. Kidney sludge may not be painful passing out the ureter, but it is nevertheless deadly over time as it slowly chokes off kidney function nephron by nephron.

How extensive is the problem? **Virtually, every living person has some degree of sludge build up and some loss of kidney function over time.** The only question is how much. Does it reach the point where it causes painful kidney stones to form or the point where it chokes off a critical mass of kidney tissue, ultimately leading to kidney failure.

It should be noted that although kidney stones and gallstones are not identical, the mechanisms involved in their formation are remarkably similar. This means that the same formulas used for eliminating kidney sludge and kidney stones will also help remove gallstones – and for that matter, even help with removing pancreatic sludge and arthritic calcium deposits in joints.

Kidney failure occurs when the kidneys are no longer able to keep the blood balanced. In acute kidney failure, symptoms include swelling, drowsiness, and irregular heartbeat. In chronic kidney failure, symptoms include fatigue, loss of appetite, headaches, cramps and thirst.

In addition to sludge, the other major kidney problems are connected to infection, inflammation, and direct damage to the protein that makes up the kidney tissue as a result of high sugar and high insulin levels.

A growing epidemic

The National Kidney and Urologic Diseases Information Clearinghouse estimates that each year, nearly 100,000 Americans are newly diagnosed with kidney failure. More than 100,000 currently have End Stage Renal Disease (ESRD) due to diabetes, and **an astounding 7.7 million have physiological evidence of chronic kidney disease.** (1) According to the U.S. Health and Human Services Agency for Healthcare Research and Quality, an estimated 650,000 Americans will have kidney failure by 2010 and will require renal replacement therapy, either ongoing renal dialysis or a kidney transplant. (2) Without one of these therapies, ESRD is fatal. Yikes!

Fortunately, it's good to know there are ways to keep your kidneys healthy to avoid going down that road.

Taking care of your kidneys

Paramount to good care of the kidneys is reducing the toxic load they have to deal with, especially proteins and chemical contaminants which can build up in the kidneys, slowing their function, increasing acidity and raising blood pressure. So, consider lightening the diet—instead of eating meat every day, try going vegetarian for a day or so a week. A vegetable/fruit-based diet allows the body system to alkalinize via the kidneys, lowering blood pressure, and contributing to a sense of well-being. Also, drinking enough water so that the urine is a light color of yellow. A whole lot of water is not necessarily good for the kidneys, and it is always better to drink small amounts of water throughout the day, rather than gulping down a quart or two because you're thirsty. This just creates kidney stress.

The regular use of a kidney cleansing and rebuilding formula is now mandatory considering the stresses we put our kidneys under thanks to our "modern" lifestyles. A good kidney formula/s will include most of the following properties and ingredients.

What the formula needs to do

- Anti-lithic (stone breaking)
- Diuretic (water removing)
- Antiseptic (infection killing)
- Anti-nephrotoxic and anti-hepatotoxic
- Soothing to urinary tract tissue
- Anti-inflammatory
- Stimulating to renal tissue

A note on stones

Different stones in the body have different chemical make-ups.

For example, gallstones are primarily formed from cholesterol, bile salts, and proteins. The more protein, the harder the stones. Think of it like the protein used to make fingernails. Incidentally, this protein primarily comes from the lining of the gallbladder. In other words, although stones get their start in the liver, they turn problematic in the gallbladder – which is why removing the gallbladder gets rid of symptoms, but not necessarily the underlying problem, which starts in the liver.

Pancreatic stones are formed from fatty acids, calcium, and proteins.

And kidney stones themselves vary significantly. There are four types.

- **Calcium stones** are composed of calcium that is chemically bound to oxalate (calcium oxalate) or phosphate (calcium phosphate).
- **Uric acid stones.** If the acid level in the urine is high or too much acid is excreted, the uric acid may not dissolve and uric acid stones may form. **Struvite or infection stones** develop when a urinary tract infection alters the chemical balance of the urine causing stones to form from ammonium, magnesium, phosphate (aka struvite).
- **Cysteine stones.** Some people inherit a rare condition that results in large amounts of cystine in the urine, which causes the formation of cystine stones that are difficult to treat.

The important thing to understand is that although all of the above types of stones have different chemical compositions, most of them can be dissolved by the right combination of herbs in a single formula.

What to look for in a formula

Chanca piedra (*Phyllanthus niruri*)

For a number of years now, I have recommended using chanca piedra before liver detoxing to soften gallstones before trying to pass them during the detox. Chanca piedra works equally well on gallstones, kidney stones, and kidney sludge. In fact, the name chanca piedra, as it is known in Peru, comes from its effect on kidney stones and gallstones. The literal translation is "stone breaker." It effectively softens both kidney stones and gallstones for easy passage out of the body. It is also renowned for its diuretic qualities and has been shown effective at helping relieve edema and urine retention. It also works as an anti-inflammatory agent in the kidneys and as an antihepatotoxic in the liver. That is to say, it counters the effects of toxins in the liver.

Hydrangea root (*Hydrangea Arborescens*)

The most common use for hydrangea is for the kidneys and bladder because of its effective diuretic property which helps increase the flow of urine. This removes impurities from the system and lessens the likelihood of infection along the entire urinary tract, which includes the kidneys, bladder, prostate (in men) and urethra. Hydrangea, like chanca piedra, is also considered an anti-lithic herb, which prevents stones or gravel from forming in the kidneys and bladder. As an anti-lithic herb, it can also assist the body in removing stones and gravel from these organs. This was a primary use of hydrangea by Native Americans.

Like most diuretic herbs, hydrangea is an excellent choice for treating inflamed or enlarged prostate glands. It is commonly combined with horsetail for this purpose. Maintaining healthy urine flow keeps the prostate less likely to constrict around the urethra, which prevents stagnant urine from causing more infection. This can also reduce inflammation by eliminating impurities from the prostate.

A scientific study published in Bioscience, Biotechnology, and Biochemistry in 2003 noted that hydrangea root extracts have greater antioxidant power in liver tissue than milk thistle and turmeric combined. The findings of Japanese researchers amplify observations of nineteenth-century American physicians who used hydrangea primarily as a treatment for "kidney gravel," small stones in the kidneys that could be passed with a minimum of pain after treatment with the herb. Physicians of the time also used hydrangea as a treatment for chronic chest pain caused by bronchitis. Hydrangea root powder has a greater diuretic effect than other preparations of the herb, but it has less of an effect on pain.

Gravel root (*Eupatorium purpureum*)

Like chanca piedra and hydrangea, gravel root also exhibits both diuretic and anti-lithic properties. Used primarily for kidney stones or gravel (which accounts for its name), it also helps with cystitis, dysuria, urethritis, and pelvic inflammatory disease. It can also play a role in the systemic treatment of rheumatism and gout as it encourages excretion of excess uric acid. And finally, it tones the reproductive tract and is used to treat inflammation of the prostate.

Marshmallow root (*Althaea Officinalis*)

Marshmallow's highest medicinal acclaim is as a demulcent. Internally it has a soothing effect on inflamed and irritated tissues of the alimentary canal, and urinary and respiratory organs. It aids in the passage of kidney stones and is used in combination with other diuretic herbs for kidney treatments which assist in the release of gravel and stones. It works very well for urinary problems. Marshmallow has factors which combine with and eliminate toxins, helping the body to cleanse. This makes marshmallow an excellent herb to add to other formulas to help neutralize toxins that are the causative factors of arthritis. Marshmallow is also very soothing to any sore or inflamed part(s) of the body. As well as the urinary tract, this herb will soothe an irritated digestive tract and help with diarrhea or dysentery.

Juniper berry (*Juniperus communis*)

Juniper Berries are used to treat infections, especially within the urinary tract, bladder, kidneys, and prostate. Their antiseptic properties help remove waste and acidic toxins from the body, stimulating a fighting action against bacterial and yeast infections. Juniper Berries also help increase the flow of digestive fluids, improving digestion and eliminating gas and stomach cramping. As a diuretic, Juniper Berries eliminate excess water retention contributing to weight loss. Juniper Berries' anti-inflammatory properties are ideal for relieving pain and inflammation related to rheumatism and arthritis. In addition, Juniper Berries are beneficial in reducing congestion, as well as treating asthma and colds. Juniper Berries make an excellent antiseptic in conditions such as cystitis. But the essential oil present in this herb is quite stimulating to the kidney nephrons. Some texts warn that juniper oil may be a kidney irritant at higher doses, but there is no real evidence that this is the case, and the dosage in this formula is quite low. Nonetheless, people with serious kidney disease probably shouldn't take juniper.

Contemporary herbalists primarily use juniper as a diuretic ("water pill") component of herbal formulas designed to treat bladder infections. The volatile oils of juniper reportedly increase the rate of kidney filtration, thereby increasing urine flow and perhaps helping to "wash out" offending bacteria. The volatile oils, particularly terpinen-4-ol, may cause an increase in urine volume. According to some sources, juniper increases urine volume without a loss of electrolytes such as potassium. It is recommended by the German Commission E for kidney ailments.

Corn silk *(Maydis stigma)*

Corn silk is a soothing diuretic and works as an excellent remedy for urinary conditions such as retained urine, burning urine, kidney stones, bladder infections, gonorrhea, and as a lymphatic system cleanser. Corn Silk is used to treat bladder infections, kidney stones, infections of the prostate gland, and urinary infections.

Uva ursi *(Arctosyaphylos uva ursi)*

The chief constituent of Uva Ursi is a glycoside called arbutin. This is what is responsible for its diuretic action. During its excretion arbutin produces an antiseptic effect on the urinary mucous membrane and can therefore help eliminate urinary tract infections. Tannic acid is also contained in the leaves. This herb also helps to keep the pH balance of urine from being too acid. It actually strengthens the lining of the urinary tract and helps to relieve any inflammation in the system. It has a direct sedative effect on the bladder walls. Allantoin, also found in Uva Ursi spurs the healing of wounds. For chronic inflammation of the bladder or kidneys Uva Ursi has no equal. Two studies report that urine from individuals given uva ursi is active against the most commonly involved bacteria in bladder and urinary tract infection.

This study supports the results of a double blind study of 57 women with recurrent cystitis. After one year, the placebo group had 20% incidence of recurring cystitis, whereas the uva ursi group had no recurring infection.

In addition, it has anti-lithic properties that help in dissolving crystals not just in the kidneys, but throughout the body as well. It has, therefore, been used for arthritis and other painful joint problems.

Parsley root (*Petroselinum crispum*)

An important diuretic, parsley root also helps clear uric acid from the urinary tract and helps dissolve and expel gallstones and gravel – and prevent their future formation. It also inhibits the secretion of histamine and is therefore useful in treating hives and relieving other allergy symptoms. A decoction of parsley root can help eliminate bloating and reduce weight by eliminating excess water gain. Note: the German Commission E, an advisory panel on herbal medicines, has approved parsley for use in the prevention and treatment of kidney stones.

Agrimony (Agrimonia eupatoria)

Agrimony is one of the most frequently used herbal supplements for kidney stones. Primarily because of its high silica content, it can help get rid of kidney stones in a matter of weeks. Urinary incontinence, cystitis and other disorders of this system may also be treated with Agrimony.

Dandelion leaf (*Taraxacum officinale*)

Dandelion leaves and roots have been used for centuries to treat liver, gall bladder, kidney, and joint problems. In some countries, Dandelion is considered a blood purifier and is used for ailments such as eczema and cancer. It has also been used to treat poor digestion, water retention, and diseases of the liver such as hepatitis.

Dandelion leaf is also a good natural source of potassium, and will replenish any potassium that may be lost due to the diuretic action of the other herbs in this formula.

Studies show beneficial effects of dandelion on reducing urinary tract gravel, attributed to disinfectant action and possibly the presence of saponins. Dandelion has also been used traditionally to treat respiratory disorders. Dr. James Duke notes in his book, The Green Pharmacy, that numerous clinical trials have demonstrated the efficacy of dandelion leaves and root for treating pneumonia, bronchitis and upper respiratory infections. Dr. Duke recommends drinking the juice that remains after the greens have been cooked. The German Pharmacopoeia lists dandelion leaf and root for treating gastrointestinal complaints stemming from bile deficiency, as well as to stimulate appetite and diuresis. Dandelion was also used in folk medicine to ease painful joint and bone conditions. The tea reduces water retention and is considered a traditional blood purifier. The diuretic effect is also useful for reducing swelling.

Horsetail (*Equisetum arvense*)

Horsetail has not been extensively studied in people, but professional herbalists recognize that the herb has diuretic (promotes the excretion of urine) properties that may be useful for the following health problems:

- Urinary tract infections
- Kidney stones

Orange peel

Limonene and flavonoids found in orange peel seem to have anti-carcinogenic properties. They can block the carcinogenesis by acting as a blocking agent. Studies have shown that limonin and limonene can induce the enzyme activity of glutathione S-transferase, which is an important detoxifying enzyme.

In addition, orange peel has antiseptic, bactericidal, and fungicidal properties.

Peppermint (*Mentha piperita*)

Peppermint has a relaxing effect on the muscles of the digestive and urinary system. It is useful for treating spasm problems in the urinary tract. It also has strong antibacterial and anti-fungal properties which help rid the kidneys of bacteria.

Three double-blind trials found that enteric-coated peppermint oil reduced the pain associated with intestinal spasms, commonly experienced in IBS.

Goldenrod (*Solidago virguarea*)

Goldenrod is used as an aquaretic agent, meaning that it promotes the loss of water from the body (as compared to a diuretic, which promotes the loss of both water and electrolytes such as salt). It is used frequently in Europe to treat urinary tract inflammation and to prevent or treat kidney stones. In fact, goldenrod has received official recognition in Germany for its effectiveness in getting rid of kidney stones, and it is commonly found in teas to help "flush out" kidney stones and stop inflammatory diseases of the urinary tract. Goldenrod is said to wash out bacteria and kidney stones by increasing the flow of urine, and also, soothe inflamed tissues and calm muscle spasms in the urinary tract. It isn't used as a cure in itself, but rather as an adjunct to other, more definitive treatments such as (in the case of bladder infections) antibiotics.

Several studies have found that goldenrod does in fact increase urine flow.

Who should use this formula and when

Since everyone accumulates sludge in their kidneys and livers, everyone is a candidate for regular use of this formula. Even people who have had their gallbladders removed will benefit. Regular softening and flushing of stones and gravel will keep your kidneys, liver, and gallbladder functioning at optimum levels and, more importantly, keep areas of those organs from choking to death and becoming non-functional. The sooner you start in life the better, but certainly the older you get, the more mandatory regular use becomes. And as for anyone already suffering from painful kidney stones or gallstones, this formula can be a godsend. Whereas medical doctors can offer only surgery or expensive lithotripsy procedures (which are also not without risk), this formula offers a safe, highly effective alternative – that can work with remarkable speed. Painful kidney stones and gallstones can usually soften enough for easy passage in as little as 2-8 days. And regular use of the formula can prevent any recurrence.

How to use

Simple

Use 4-8 droppers in diluted juice three times a day until bottle is gone.

Better

Take 4 ounces of this formula and mix with a quart of fresh squeezed apple juice (not bottled) and a quart of water. Drink a pint each day over 4 days.

For most people, doing this program twice a year should be enough to keep the kidneys functioning properly. An ideal time to do this program is shortly before doing a liver detox. Again, the same herbs that soften kidney stones for easy passage will also soften gallbladder stones. Using this formula shortly before doing the liver detox will greatly reduce the likelihood of discomfort when doing the liver detox.

For those who have a predilection to getting kidney stones or gallstones, this program can be done once a month to minimize the chances of any future occurrence.

If you have currently existing painful kidney or gallstones, you probably will want to mix up two batches and drink it for 8 straight days.

Do not do more than once a month on a regular basis as the diuretic effect may deplete the body of essential water-soluble vitamins and minerals over time.

Note: If using in preparation for the liver detox, make sure you use within 30 days of starting the detox so the gallstones don't get a chance to reharden before flushing.

Warning: The diuretic effects of this formula may enhance the toxic effects of certain medications, such as digoxin (used to treat congestive heart failure), phenytoin (for seizures), anticoagulants, and others. For this reason, people taking prescription medications should not use this formula without first consulting a health care provider. Also, anyone with severe kidney problems should not use this formula without first consulting their physician.

Don't Stop Drinking Water

So now it's water. If you are to believe what the media has been saying in the past, there are no health benefits to drinking water. Drinking water or cola are pretty much the same thing. And dehydration is a myth.

Really?

No, not really. As usual, the media got the story all wrong — and, as it turns out, even the accurate story is much less than it seems. In this issue of the newsletter, we'll see how the media once again lost the truth by attempting to reduce science to a sound bite and how research that the sound bite is based on is pretty much meaningless. Then we'll wrap things up with a discussion of what you really need to know about water.

The media...again

If you saw the headlines, you're probably thinking that water is about to be pulled from the market and anyone who sold it was about to be arrested for running one of the greatest consumer scams of all time.

- Study pours cold water on drinking eight glasses a day
- Water Study Disproves 8 Glass Rule
- Extra water is no help, it only stretches your bladder: study
- Zero Health Benefit from Drinking Extra Water

- Need For 8 Glasses of Water A Day 'A Myth' Say Researchers
- Study: Skip the Water, Have a Soda Instead

Read the headlines and there can be no mistake. A scientific study conducted by Drs. Negoianu and Goldfarb has proven that there are no health benefits to drinking 8 glasses of water a day! But there is little truth to the headlines. The media's reporting on the "study" is wrong on a number of counts.

- First, it was not a study at all — merely a cursory examination of pre-existing scientific literature. No new ground was broken here, just a reinterpretation of older reviews and studies — only one of which specifically looked at drinking 8 glasses of water a day. The others involved indirect inference. Or to look at it another way, this report, just published in the *Journal of the American Society of Nephrology*, would be disallowed in a court of law as "hearsay" evidence.
- But more to the point, contrary to what the headlines say, the report in question never actually says that drinking 8 glasses of water a day provides no health benefits — merely that there is not yet any clear proof that it does. To quote, "To summarize the conclusions of other, more exhaustive reviews: There is no clear evidence of benefit from drinking increased amounts of water. Although we wish we could demolish all of the urban myths found on the Internet regarding the benefits of supplemental water ingestion, **we concede there is also no clear evidence of lack of benefit. In fact, there is simply a lack of evidence in general.**"
- And finally, the study never actually says that drinking soda is the same as drinking water. Yes, some of the other studies that this study refers to make that claim — but not this study. In other words, headlines above such as "Study: Skip the Water, have a Soda Instead" are nothing more than inaccurate media sound bites.

In summary, we can throw out the headlines and stories as found in the media. Now to be fair, as advertising revenues have dropped, newspapers and television networks all over the world have dramatically cut their reporting staffs to save money — and for the most part now have to function as reporters and transcribers of news, rather than as investigative journalists. In other words, not one of the media reports actually looked beyond the press release associated with the review. That said, we're still left with the question when it comes to drinking water, "What then did Drs. Negoianu and Goldfarb actually say in their review?"

The 8 glasses of water review

They begin their review by examining a handful of studies that support the drinking of more water and dismiss them all in a single brushstroke. To quote:

"Of course, these studies suffered from weaknesses typical of epidemiologic and retrospective case-control data: Are people sick because they drink less, or are they drinking less because they are sick?"

It seems that Negoianu and Goldfarb are starting with a fundamental premise that any existing study that supports the use of water is fundamentally flawed and should not be considered in drawing any conclusions. But they also seem to be starting with the equally questionable premise that almost any study that negates the value of drinking 8 glasses of water is correct ipso facto and should be highly valued. These are interesting assumptions since they pretty much guarantee your conclusion before you even started. With that in mind, let's take a look at one of the studies they believe worthy of inclusion.

At the top of their list is the 2002 Valtin study that they describe as an "exceedingly thorough review of this subject." High praise, indeed! So, what exactly is this benchmark study? Well, first surprise, it's not a study at all. Like the Negoianu and Goldfarb review, it too is a review of previous studies. And like the Negoianu and Goldfarb review, it too is based on some "interesting" assumptions.

For example, Dr. Valtin announces that just counting water intake in his review is not good enough. "The concept I have in mind is daily intake of drinking fluid (as distinct from fluid in solid food) meaning all drinking fluids, including tap water and bottled water, coffee, tea, soft drinks, milk, juices, and possibly even beer in moderation."

Excuse me! As a study of the health benefits of drinking 8 glasses of water a day, you can pretty much toss this review out from the get-go. Not all fluids are the same. If you think so, try washing your clothes in beer and soda. But then again, perhaps it was the happy inclusion of beer and soda that led Drs. Negoianu and Goldfarb to think so highly of Valtin's "exceedingly thorough review."

Yes, I understand. Dr. Valtin would disagree with me. He cites the Grandjean study, which concluded that there is no significant difference between water, soda, coffee, beer, etc.when it comes to hydration. And yes, that's possibly true if you limit your discussion to the volume of fluids entering and leaving the body; but that doesn't mean that there's no difference. What those liquids contain when they enter the body — and when they leave the body — are not necessarily the same for all liquids, regardless of volume. The Grandjean study, for example, didn't consider the effects in his other "drinking fluids" of sugar (promotes diabetes), artificial sweeteners (they make you fat and give you cancer), phosphoric acid (causes osteoporosis), or caffeine (increases the risk of spontaneous abortion) on the body. Drinking water and soda are not the same thing. There really are differences in terms of health. So much for the Grandjean study.

Is there any evidence that drinking more than the minimum amount of water is beneficial?

As it turns out, there's quite a bit. Here is just a sampling.

- The more water you drink, the less your chances of developing kidney stones
- Higher water consumption has been associated with lower rates of urinary cancer
- A relationship between high water intake and lower colon cancer risk
- A higher intake of water reduces the incidence of heart attacks

That said, Drs. Negoianu and Goldfarb were correct when they stated that **there is simply a lack of evidence in general.** As they and Dr. Valtin all found, there are quite simply no actual studies that focus on the overall benefits of drinking 8 glasses of water a day. All conclusions, at the moment, are based on inference from studies that were focused on other agendas — and the people doing the inferring have no understanding or affinity for the value of complementary health.

But what about the anecdotal evidence on drinking water?

However, let's not ignore anecdotal evidence. Just because researchers haven't proven the benefits of a particular alternative health treatment yet, doesn't mean it's not valid. Consider all of the fruits and plants whose benefits were touted for centuries without proof — only to be found to contain amazingly beneficial phytochemicals in the last few years. Also, consider all of the herbs used by healers since the dawn of man that ultimately became the basis for some of the world's most powerful drugs. We're talking about plants which became drugs such as Chinese star anise, which was the basis for Tamiflu, saw palmetto for Proscar, Pacific yew for Tamoxifen, and foxglove for Digitalis — just to name a few.

And finally, let's not discount the anecdotal evidence of millions of people around the world who testify to better health and greater vitality when they increase their consumption of water. Even if it is a placebo effect, it's still a positive effect, and water is a whole lot cheaper than the placebo effect achieved by "approved" medical procedures such as angioplasty or mainstream drugs such as Zetia and Vytorin.

But enough! I could go on ripping through these studies pointing out their deficiencies ad infinitum. But there's no need; the point has been made. Time to move on and talk briefly about the quality and quantity of water you need — at least as we understand it at this time.

Not all water is the same.

To put it simply, you want the purest water you can get that also contains essential trace minerals and that is pH optimized and, in a form, that your body can most readily utilize. In that regard, not all water is the same.

- Avoid chlorine and chloramines in your water. They are known carcinogens and kill all beneficial bacteria.
- Avoid fluoride in your water. It makes your bones weaker, encourages the deposit of aluminum in the brain, and lowers immune levels throughout the body.
- Drink water with optimized molecular groupings to improve cellular transport. There are many ways this can be accomplished, but applying a magnetic field to the water certainly works, and it's inexpensive. The interesting thing is that plants, which are not subject to the placebo effect, grow much better on water subjected to a magnetic field.
- Drink water that has an alkaline pH. As detailed in Chapter 13 of ***Lessons from the Miracle Doctors,*** maintaining a blood pH of around 7.45, without compromising the pH of the surrounding tissue, is vital. This requires the presence of minerals since pure distilled water has a neutral pH but turns slightly acid over time as it absorbs carbon dioxide from the air, thus forming carbonic acid.

How much water do we need?

In advanced societies, thinking that tea, coffee, alcohol, soda pop, or other forms of manufactured beverages are desirable substitutes for the purely natural water needs of the daily "stressed" body is a common, but potentially deadly, mistake. Water is **the** solvent in our bodies, and as such, it regulates all the functions of our bodies, including the action of all the solids dissolved in the water. In fact, every function of the body is monitored and pegged to the efficient flow of water. Think for a moment of just a few of the functions that water regulates:

- The movement of blood
- The transport of nutrients into our cells
- The movement of waste out of our cells
- The flow of lymph fluid
- The movement of nerve impulses through our nerves
- The movement of hormones throughout our bodies
- The functioning of our brains

Understand, we can function quite well and for quite a long time without sufficient water. The body quickly adapts and starts extracting more water from your stools for example. The kidneys flush less water to retain the limited supply you have. In fact, there are some health experts who claim that your body does quite well on 2 glasses of any kind of fluid a day — plus the water found in the food you eat. **But these experts confuse adaptation with health. Adaptation leads to compromise, which leads to diminished health over time.**

Look, ultimately it may be proven that drinking more than 2 glasses of water a day has no health benefits, but that day has not arrived yet — and the Negoianu, Goldfarb review does not bring it any closer. It's bad science, bad reporting by the press, and shoddy peer review by the Journal of the *American Society of Nephrology*. Therefore, until it is actually proven otherwise, keep targeting between 64 and 96 ounces of pure water a day. Pure, fresh (not bottled or canned) fruit and vegetable juices may be substituted for some of this quantity — as may limited quantities of non-diuretic herbal teas (without sugar). In general, however, pure water is the key.

Ref: Date: 08/15/2007 DR Jon Barron
Ref: NATURE. Ikezoe, N. Hirota, J. Nakagawa and K. Kitazawa, Making water levitate, Nature 393 (1998) 749-750).

Emotions and Health

Good emotional health is very underrated in today's times. Though alternative medicine and even common belief dictates that mental, emotional, physical, and spiritual well-being are intertwined and what affects one component affects the others, too many people ignore their emotional health. In the pursuit of material security and the struggles to keep up with the pressures of a fast-paced life, individuals end up getting extremely stressed, sapped, and even depressed.

Negative emotions, including the ones we take for granted, such as anxiety, fear, frustration, envy, and doubt can affect your health to a great degree. Certain occurrences in life, such as getting fired from the job, experiencing monetary problems, going through a tumultuous marriage, or coping with the death of a loved one, can wreak havoc on one's mental and emotional state and in turn take a toll on the body.

If that sounds far-fetched, but let's shed light on the numerous health hazards of being burdened with negative emotions.

How Emotions Affect the Body

Unknown to many, the human body reacts to the way we feel and think. For instance, extreme stress has been known to cause gastric ulcers and high blood pressure even in people who do not have a family or past history of these conditions. Such physical signs are a way of telling us that we need to sit up, take notice, and turn our lives around for the better.

The most common signs of negative emotion-induced conditions include:

- Excessive tiredness
- Stomach problems
- Significant weight loss or weight gain
- Back and neck problems
- Insomnia
- Sexual dysfunction
- Breathing problems
- Change in appetite
- Hampered immunity

Negative emotions have even been linked to premature death. For instance, in a study conducted by researchers on over 7000 subjects over a span of four decades, it was noted that optimists are more likely to live longer lives than pessimists. What really stood out was the fact that the individuals who were pessimistic in their youth were 42 percent more susceptible to a faster death than their counterparts- a figure that would indeed shock many. Optimism is linked to fewer incidences of depression and stress and a healthy lifestyle and body as a result.

A disturbed frame of mind and undesirable emotions can also prevent one from ensuring that he/she puts his/her health above all else. When a person is anxious, fearful, depressed, or frustrated, following a balanced diet, getting adequate sleep, and exercising on a regular basis takes a backseat. Such emotions also trigger addictive tendencies such as excess smoking, drinking, eating, and even drug abuse – all of which ultimately have a detrimental effect on physical well-being.

Certain Emotions Affect Certain Organs

Have you been experiencing a downward spiral in your emotional well-being and a consequent effect somewhere in your body in the form of pain or discomfort? The truth is that particular emotions have been known to 'target' select bodily systems:

- **Impatience and hate** can affect intestinal and heart health, and the most common symptoms are palpitations, chest pain, and hypertension
- **Depression and melancholy** can affect the large intestine, skin and lungs, the common symptoms of which are constipation, low blood oxygen count, and breathing difficulties
- **Envy, frustration, and anger** have a negative effect on the eyes, gall bladder, and liver. The common symptoms include hampered detoxification due to stagnant blood in the liver, excess cholesterol, and poor digestion due to imbalanced bile production
- **Fear** affects the urinary bladder, kidneys, and ears, and the most common symptoms are poor sexual stamina, disorders of the nervous system, excess acid production in the body, and abdominal knots
- **Mistrust, anxiety, and worry** can lead to poor digestion and difficulty with regard to waste elimination. These emotions usually have a negative effect on stomach, spleen, and pancreatic health

Living a Better Life

If you are one of the many people plagued by negative emotions to ill health, you need to adopt certain coping mechanisms and tips to get your well-being back on track. For one, modes of relaxation like walking, reading, listening to music, doing yoga, and meditating can work wonders in helping you take a break from your hectic lifestyle or routine.

Overanalyzing situations and emotions can also lead to unnecessary worry and the secretion of stress chemicals. Make it a point to exercise every day to cope better with negative emotions. You must also stop harping on the past if you want to look forward to a healthy future.

Express yourself instead of bottling everything up inside. If you are unable to open up to friends and family, do so to a counselor, doctor, religious advisor, and so on. Ensure that you have social support and maintain a journal if required.

Herbs for Hair Loss and Color

Hair loss is an issue in a wide range of age groups. Although many think that hair loss is just for the elderly, this simply isn't true. In fact, hair loss can affect some even at high school ages where embarrassment can reach at its peak.

In Chinese Medicine the hair is connected with the Kidney. Also, since the hair is often considered a 'sprouting of abundance', if you will, the hair has a strong connection to the Chinese Medicine reflection of blood and the abundance of blood in the body. These two characteristics are important in choosing internal medicinals that are helpful in treating hair loss.

Another issue that many people are trying to get rid of is grey hair. In modern times most, people utilize hair dye and chemicals including bleach. Obviously, these haven't been around as long (and some choose to take the route of not using chemicals) instead herbs have been used and believe it or not it is internal medicine instead of external application that has dominated this game.

The most famous, and dated, use of herbs has been the long use of *longevity herbs* for the Emperor of china. With long flowing black hair and status to maintain they used herbs internally to keep the hair black and herbs externally for keeping the skin light. Also, these herbs are good for supplementing the kidneys and have a positive impact on blood building.

These herbs are known for good effects with **hair growth and keeping a full head of hair**:

He Shou Wu: He Shou Wu is often referred to as Fo-Ti as well. He Shou Wu utilizes all the acts of 'longevity' by strengthening the Kidney. He Shou Wu is used for hair growth, hair darkening, and blood building. It is a good herb for longevity and long-term use. All of these attributes are linked to the long life you are able to have with taking Fo-Ti.

Gotu Kola: Main revitalizing herb for the nerves and brain cells. It is also a powerful blood purifier and helps rebuild energy reserves. Contains asiaticoside which stimulates hair and nail growth, increases development of blood vessels into connective tissue, increases tensile integrity of the dermis, exerts a balancing effect on connective tissue.

Sage: Sage reduces excess secretions, stops sweating, dries up excess mucus from the nose and lungs and salivation, dries up sores and ulcers and stops bleeding. It is great for the brain and nervous system and promotes hair growth. It also combines well with Gotu Kola.

Foxglove Root: comes in prepared (Shu) and non-prepared (Sheng) forms. Many prefer the prepared version of this herb to use as more of a tonic for darkening the hair and eliminating grey.

You can also add these herbs along with herbs like Bu Gu Zhi to a tincture and apply a small amount externally with shampoo daily. These herbs are never able to single out one function so they are also useful for hair loss as well. Side effects will also include moistened skin, better sleep, improved vision, and more energy. A side effect many may welcome.

These are also a few herbs that have been helping **hair loss in women** for thousands of years.

Hemp Seed: The oils of the hemp seed are used for many purposes in Chinese Medicine and they prove to be very reliable. Hemp seed can be pounded or ground and applied directly to the scalp and left for a while and then washed away.

Platycladus: has volatile oils in it that are known to be healthy to scalp health, and we know is healthy to skin. It can be made into a tincture or cooked like a decoction and applied to the scalp daily. It is effective for hair loss and itchy scalp, so it has a bit of a dual purpose!

Top 10 Genetically Modified Foods to Avoid

Genetically modified foods (GMO) are those foods that are primarily derived from genetically modified organisms. These genetically derived organisms have undergone specific changes to their DNA using genetic engineering techniques that exploit the natural forms of gene transfer.

Are GMO's Safe for You?

Genetically modified foods are subject to debate, ever since they were put in the market in 1996. Many critics object to GM foods due to safety issues and many other ecological and economical concerns. However, due to lack of labeling, the consumers barely know what products are genetically modified and which ones are suitable for use. Therefore, the use of GMO's continues.

Here, is the list of **top 10 foods** that have been genetically modified

- **Corn:** According to FDA, genetically modified corn is now available for human use. However, it has been found that this kind of genetically modified corn was meant to create an insecticide, which when consumed could lead to problems with fertility.

- **Soy:** GM soy has been used for a variety of soy products including soy flour, soy beverages, and soybean oil. It is known that when hamsters were fed with the GM variety of soy, they showed increased mortality rate. Imagine this could happen to humans too!
- **Cotton:** GM cotton was designed to resist pesticides. While Chinese agriculture confirmed that genetically modified corn proved excellent for keeping pests away from the corn fields, many Indian cotton farmers have reported to have suffered from rashes due to exposure to GM cotton.
- **Papaya:** In 1999, Hawaiian Papaya was introduced which was genetically modified to resist papaya ringspot virus. Papaya ringspot virus (PRSV) is considered to hamper the production of papaya, which is why, transgenic papaya is now being developed in different parts of the world including countries like Thailand, Jamaica, Brazil, and Venezuela.
- **Rice:** Rice is a staple food for many countries in Asia. A genetically modified variety of rice has been introduced that is rich in Vitamin A. In a China Daily article, it was reported that GM rice posed potential health, economic and environment problems. GM rice has a tendency to develop allergic reactions, and there is an increased possibility of gene transfer due to GM rice.
- **Tomatoes:** In order to improve the shelf life of tomatoes, naturally grown tomatoes are being genetically modified too. GM tomatoes do not rot easily in transfers and exports. However, it was reported that when these tomatoes were fed to a few animal subjects, they died after sometime.
- **Rapeseed:** The GM variety of rapeseed is also known as canola, and it is popularly used in making canola oil. Today, honey can also be produced from canola. However, German food authorities confirmed that Canadian honey is heavily pollinated by GM rapeseed as most of the honey products coming from Canada contained pollen from GM rapeseed.
- **Dairy Products:** Nearly 22% of the cows in United States are injected with genetically modified bovine growth hormone (rbGH)

for increased milk production. However, it has been reported that milk from those cows that have been treated with rbGH contained a high amount of IGF-1 (insulin growth factors-1), which has been found to cause breast cancer.

- **Potatoes:** GM potatoes are genetically engineered. It has been reported that mice fed with genetically modified potatoes contained high amounts of toxins in their system. Needless to say, GM potatoes pose a threat to human health, as well.
- **Peas:** There is a wide variety of GM peas available in the market. However, it has been known that genetically modified peas harm the immune system and is dangerous for human consumption. In fact, when a kidney bean gene was combined with that of peas, a protein was generated that could well function to reduce pests.

Genetically modified foods have often been associated with some of the strangest diseases including Morgellon's disease, a condition that involves symptoms like the feeling of crawling black speckled materials under the skin. Many patients having this disease have also reported short term memory loss, change in vision and mental confusion.

American Academy of Environmental Medicine (AAEM) has been warning use of GM foods and how these genetically modified foods are a threat to human health. However, the production and sale of GMO's continues and it is left to consumers to decide whether it is suitable for consumption or not!

Next time you go to your supermarket for buying any of the above food items, do yourself a favor – avoid buying GM foods and choose the natural variety instead.

Baked Goods Contain Ingredient that Causes Cancer

Baked goods are one of the most popular foods amongst people, because of their amazing taste and health benefits. People love to eat bread with their meals – be it white, wheat or honey oats. But there is a hidden danger that you might not know about.

Obesity is one of the major causes of many diseases including heart attack, and hence people have started opting for a healthier lifestyle by avoiding junk food. But who would know that baked goods that are sold in US can cause something even deadlier than heart disease? Yes, most of the baked goods sold in US contain potassium bromate that causes cancer.

According to a research conducted by American Agency for Research on Cancer (IARC) potassium bromate used in baked goods can cause cancer.

What is Potassium Bromate?

Potassium bromate is an oxidizing agent and is used in baked goods as it strengthens the dough and makes the finished product look great. In a 1982 research, it was revealed that potassium bromate is used in baking goods because it gives higher rising properties that results in a fluffy and light bread. It was also found that this chemical is dangerous for consumption and causes cancer. Tests done on rats and mice confirmed that it can cause tumor in kidney and other organs. The publication of this research resulted in the ban of potassium bromate in United Kingdom, Canada and Australia but not in USA.

Ban Potassium Bromate in US

Despite of the dangerous nature of potassium bromate, it is still not banned in US, and most bakers are using it. Why? This is because it helps in raising the flour, hence decreasing the baking time and saving energy.

The Center of Science in Public Interest petitioned FDA to ban the use of this ingredient, but it has been unable to do so, because of a loophole in the American food regulation which they are unwilling to change. The FDA (Food and drug administration) in US urged bakers to stop using potassium bromate willingly when research indicated that is responsible for causing cancer in human. The FDA in an action to limit the usage of potassium bromate has asked the bakers in California to indicate on the goods that it contains bromated flour; hence this has caused the bakers to stop using it.

How to Make Baked Goods with Bromated Flour?

Well, it's not that bakery items cannot be made without bromated flour; there are many bakers who have never used it and still have the best products and flour. King Arthur flour mill is a prime example, their flour is free of potassium bromate and is used by renowned bakers worldwide to make those delicious delicacies. Potassium bromate is a core ingredient in baked product but can easily be replaced; all it will require is just a bit of more time and energy. Making delicious baked goods without bromated flour requires a slight shift in the mixing process and a bit more time for baking as the rising time of the bakery increases.

Note to Consumers in US

Prevention is better than cure. Research by has clearly indicated that baked goods contain potassium bromate causes cancer. Hence, one should be cautious when buying bread.

A note of advice to our listeners:

- Whenever buying baked goods, always check the ingredients and if they contain potassium bromate ask for a product that is free from this ingredient.
- There are bakers who sell bromate free goodies; try finding them in your state, a little bit of effort will protect you against a deadly disease.
- If finding bromate free bread is difficult, a better option is to buy flour and make bread at home. This will help in ensuring health for the family.
- Remember potassium bromate and bromated flour are the same. So, don't let yourself be fooled by this gimmick.

According to a research published by the World Health Organization (WHO), the number of deaths caused by cancer will increase from 7.6 million in 2005 to 9 million in 2015 and approximately 12 million by 2030.

The changing global dynamics and sedentary lifestyle are common reasons for the increase in cancer patients. Keeping these statistics in mind consumer should be careful and avoid using potassium bromate and other such products that may result in cancer. Furthermore, FDA should look in to the matter more seriously, and reconsideration should be made in order to ban this and other harmful ingredients that are used in baked goods.

Health Benefits of Quinoa

Quinoa is a Powerful Vegetable Seed!

Although referred to as a grain, it is actually a seed from a vegetable related to Swiss chard, spinach and beets. Quinoa is pronounced *keen-wa* not *kwin-o-a*.

Quinoa was considered sacred by the Incas; they called it the "mother seed." The Inca civilization in South America grew it in the high altitude of the Andes. It was their staple food for 5,000 years. The Spanish conquistadors almost wiped quinoa out by making it illegal for the Indians to grow. They did not see how useful it is. Finally, in the 1980s two Americans discovered this nutrient-rich food and began growing quinoa in Colorado.

8 Health Benefits of Quinoa:

1. **High quality protein** with the nine essential amino acids, the protein balance is similar to milk. At 16.2 to 20 percent protein, it has is more protein than rice (7.5 percent), millet (9.9 percent) or wheat (14 percent).
2. **Great source of riboflavin**. Riboflavin has been shown to help reduce the frequency of attacks in migraine sufferers by improving the energy metabolism within the brain and muscle cells.

3. Inca warriors had more **stamina and quicker recovery time** by eating these quinoa seeds, making it a truly ancient **powerfood**.
4. **Antiseptic.** The saponins from quinoa are used to promote healing of skin injuries in South America.
5. **Not fattening!** Only 172 calories per 1/4 cup dry (24 of the calories from protein and only 12 from sugars, the rest are complex carbohydrates, fiber and healthy fats).
6. **Gluten-free.** Since it is not related to wheat, or even a grain, it is gluten-free.
7. **Alkaline-forming.** Although it is not strongly alkaline-forming, it is comparable to wild rice, amaranth, and sprouted grains.
8. **Smart Carb:** It is a complex carbohydrate with a low glycemic index, so it won't spike your blood sugar.

Interesting facts:

More than 200,000 pounds are gown each year in the US Rocky Mountains. Quinoa is the whitest and the sweetest tasting when grown above 12,500 feet. When it is grown at lower elevations, it is more bittersweet in taste. Quinoa thrives at altitudes of 9,000 to 13,000 feet above sea level and survives on as little as two inches of rainfall.

Use and Safety:

Quinoa, though highly nutritious, is actually coated with the toxic chemical saponin; you must rinse the quinoa thoroughly. Saponins can be challenging to the immune system and stomach. Commercial processing methods remove much of the bitter soapy saponins coating quinoa seeds, but it is best to rinse again to remove any of the powdery saponins that may remain on the seeds. Like any good foods, we need variety so do not eat it every day. A few times a week is good enough.

Although quinoa is not a commonly allergenic food and does not contain lots of purines, it does contain oxalates. This puts quinoa on the caution list for an oxalate-restricted diet.

Clean Up the Toxic Cosmetics Aisle

Take a walk down the children's products aisle at your local drug store and you'll see dozens of items – shampoo, sunscreen, bubble bath – marked "gentle," "for sensitive skin," or "no tears." These labels are there to assure parents that the personal care products we put on our children's bodies are formulated especially for kids.

Many parents assume that if a product is marketed to or for children, it must be safe.

Unfortunately, that's not the case.

Major loopholes in the law make cosmetics and body care products among the least regulated consumer products on the market today; in fact, the vast majority of the approximately 12,500 chemicals used by the $50 billion beauty industry have never been assessed for safety. It's perfectly legal for cosmetics and personal care products to contain chemical linked to cancer, reproductive and developmental harm, hormone disruption, asthma and other adverse health effects. Some of these chemicals don't even appear on product labels so even the most well-informed consumers can't protect their families.

American consumers use an average of 10 personal care products each day, resulting in exposure to more than 100 distinct chemicals, and potentially dozens of hidden ingredients. Toxic cosmetic ingredients are ending up inside our bodies, our breast milk and our babies and these chemicals also go down the drain and pollute our waterways and drinking water. Toxic exposures from personal care products add to our daily dose of hazardous chemicals from air, water, food and other consumer products.

And the cosmetics industry is now targeting tween girls with its products—girls who are hitting puberty at younger and younger ages which can contribute to their risk of developing breast cancer later in life (among other health problems).

Fortunately, for the first time in 30 years, in response to public outcry around formaldehyde in hair products and baby shampoo, mercury in face cream, and lead in lipstick Congress is paying attention to cosmetics safety.

The Safe Cosmetics Act of 2011, would give the FDA the authority and resources it needs to ensure that cosmetics are safe by: phasing out the worst chemicals in cosmetics that can cause cancer or reproductive harm; requiring companies to be transparent and honest about what's in their products; and establishing a strong safety standard to make sure decisions about ingredient safety protect the most vulnerable populations –babies, children, pregnant women and workers.

Unfortunately, the titans of the cosmetics industry are also hard at work fighting common sense laws that would keep toxic chemicals out of everything from bubble bath to lipstick.

"The Cosmetic Safety Amendments Act of 2012," a bill written by the Personal Care Products Council, a trade association that represents the big multinational cosmetic companies, was recently introduced into Congress. This is a classic Trojan horse – it may sound like a step forward on the surface but the "fine print" inside the bill would allow industry to continue placing profits over public health—putting into law the current system that allows the industry to "self-regulate" the safety of cosmetics.

So, what's a mom (or dad) to do?

A growing number of companies are paying attention to the demand for safer products. You can vote with your dollar to buy safer products for your family.

To Know which products are safe and where they score on the safety scorecard visit the website www.ewg.org.

Hidden Truth about Fluoride and its Danger

An overwhelming amount of information is building up against fluoride and its potential dangers. It has been linked to a variety of severe chronic, even acute health issues.

From drinking water to a vast number of drugs and medicines, everything around us has some percentage of fluoride. Can fluoride really wreak havoc on our health? If you want to know the answer to this question, then listen on to find out.

Fluoride is a soluble salt, not a heavy metal. There are two basic types of fluoride. **Calcium fluoride** appears naturally in underground water sources and even seawater. Enough of it can cause skeletal or dental fluorosis, which weakens bone and dental matter. But it is not nearly as toxic, nor does it negatively affect so many other health issues as **sodium fluoride**, which is added to many water supplies. This fluoride has capacity to combine and increase the potency of other toxic materials. The sodium fluoride obtained from industrial waste and added to water supplies is also already contaminated with lead, aluminum, and cadmium.

It damages the liver and kidneys, weakens the immune system, creates symptoms that mimic fibromyalgia, can cause premature birth, brain degradation, bone loss, and even cancer.

But there's another hidden danger with fluoride. It depletes iodine in the body, causing hypothyroidism and immune deficiency. It easily displaces iodine in the body, thus causing irreversible damage. While both iodine and fluoride are halogens, the latter is more reactive and toxic too. The lack of iodine or sodium in our body can cause innumerable health problems.

Iodine deficiency has been linked to thyroid disorders which can further lead to weight gain, dry skin, premature aging, depression, constipation, excessive hair loss, heart disorders, high cholesterol, and a loss of libido.

Iodine also plays a crucial role in strengthening the immune function of our bodies. Blood circulates through the thyroid gland every 17 minutes, and the iodine present in the thyroid gland kills/weakens any foreign bodies or invading organisms present in the blood. Iodine is a potent germ killer, which is why it helps in eradicating any such foreign organisms from the body, making the immune system's job easier. A lack of iodine means this critical step in the immunity function is reduced or completely eliminated, which in turn lowers your immunity.

In short, when fluoride levels increase in the body, it impacts every aspect of your health in a negative manner.

Unlike iodine, fluoride is a persistent toxin that can be stored in the body for a long time – and only half of what you ingest is excreted out, while the rest is stored in your bones and tissues. This deprives them of essential elements such as iodine.

How does fluoride get into our system? What are the sources leading to fluoride exposure?

The list of things that contain fluoride is endless: drinking water, dental hygiene products (toothpaste), breakfast cereals, concentrated juices, sodas and other aerated drinks, processed foods, some medications/drugs, and so on.

Even certain pesticides contain high levels of fluoride, which means that the environment is being flooded with fluoride by conventional agriculture.

It is high time that the amount of fluoride exposure is controlled and restored back to normal levels. In fact, in most cases, fluoridation is not necessary. As per the data collected from the World Health Organization, most Western European countries are not fluoridated and have the same level of dental decay rates as the US. Similarly, other communities from Canada, East Germany, and Finland discontinued fluoridation and actually experienced a decline in dental decay!

Here are few more reasons as to why fluoridation should be opposed:

- A journal published by the American Dental Association titled *Toxicity of Fluorides in Relation to Their Use in Dentistry* talks about the various ill-effects of fluoride and has made it clear that **fluoride is a poison**.
- Qualified scientists in multiple laboratory tests have found that even 1.0 part of fluoride added to a one million liters of water (the amount typically used in fluoridation) **acts as a potent carcinogen and mutagen**. In the US, more than 20,000 plus cancer deaths occur due to the fluoridation of water each year.
- A wide number of experiments show that that fluoride gets accumulated in the brain cells and **alters mental behavior** in a manner similar to that of a neurotoxic agent.
- Fluoride exposure is known to have a **detrimental effect on the musculoskeletal and nervous systems**, leading to muscular degeneration, neurological disorders, ligament calcification, etc.
- Excessive fluoride can actually cause discoloration and make the teeth brittle.
- It was found that the level of fluoride added to water is approx. 200 times higher than the amount found in mother's milk, which means that infants ingesting such water are exposed to serious dangers and health risks.
- Excessive fluoride consumption can also **weaken the bones** and increase the chances of hip and wrist fractures. Scientists at EPA in Washington have confirmed that the increasing numbers of

people with carpal tunnel syndrome, arthritis, joint pain, etc. are due to the mass fluoridation of drinking water.
- Fluoride exposure during pregnancy can lead to **attention deficit disorders**, learning disabilities, and other behavioral disorders in children.

Fluoride's role in causing thyroid problems is well established, and the fact that hypothyroidism affects as many as 10% of women in the United States alone does not come as a surprise. Most doctors go by the conventional approach and completely ignore the cause behind hypothyroidism, only to prescribe artificial 'thyroxin' hormone to make up for the deficiency in the body.

Is this really an answer to the ever-growing epidemic caused by fluoride exposure? No. In fact, all this has done is to create a stable, ever-expanding market for the cash cow thyroid drug companies.

One might assume that fluoride's role in suppressing thyroid and immune function is a relatively new discovery, and that the government was not aware about its harmful effects. However, the fact that fluoride was used in treating an overactive thyroid was well known, as this treatment has been in existence since the 1930s.

Fluoride is a disease-causing element and a neurotoxin that disrupts the functioning of the thyroid gland, increases the risk of cancer, weakens the bones, increases the rate of bone fractures, damages the liver and kidneys, lowers IQ, and causes dental fluorosis. The list of fluoride-related dangers is endless.

Why then, has fluoridation been an ongoing process? Why are no steps being taken to control fluoride exposure? The world is now exposed to ever-increasing doses of fluoride in toothpastes, mouth rinses, medicines, water, food, and even the air we breathe. Our environment has literally become a fluoride dumping ground, and we are still acting as mere spectators.

It is high time that the government and health officials take charge of the situation, face the various challenges posed by fluoride exposure, and take stringent measures to control fluoridation in every way possible.

Top 10 Benefits of Aloe Vera

Aloe Vera is a pretty looking plant with leaves that spread out in an offset pattern. It is basically a shrub that grows to just about 25-35 inches (60-90 cm). Aloe vera leaves have small white teeth around the edges and feel smooth on the outside and succulently spongy on the inside. When a leaf of Aloe Vera is cut open, a gel like substance is obtained. This aloe vera extract is known to contain several micronutrients including vitamin E, amino acids and enzymes that are good for skin and has many health benefits.

Aloe vera extract has been used for making various types of natural skin care products for many years. Today, it is also commercially cultivated all over the world. Apart from being used in cosmetic products, aloe vera is also used in treatment of some ailments including burns, rashes, wounds, and even bruises.

Here, are the top 10 benefits of Aloe Vera:

1. Cancer

Aloe vera contains Vitamin C and antioxidants that prevent the damage of cells. When used in combination with chemotherapy, it assists in the healing process. In many cases, it has been found to shrink tumors.

2. Obesity

Aloe is known to improve digestion. It breaks fat globules and cleanses the digestive tract and helps control obesity.

3. Diabetes

According to American Diabetes Association, diabetic patients, who took a table spoon of aloe juice twice a day, showed a significant decrease in blood sugar levels.

4. Blood Pressure

Aloe vera contains Vitamin B12, which is required for the smooth functioning of the cardiovascular system. It can also assist in preventing blockages in the arteries.

5. Detox

Aloe vera contains a cocktail of vitamins and minerals which is very good for detoxification of the body. It helps the body to deal with everyday stress.

6. Immunity

Aloe vera is full of antioxidants that fight free radicals in the body, enhancing the overall immunity system.

7. Gastric Problems

Aloe acts as a cleansing agent. When you consume aloe juice religiously for several weeks, it can effectively clear the stomach and the colon region. It also reduces the production of gastric acids and protects the lining of the stomach. As a result, gastric disorders such as constipation and irritable bowel syndrome can be controlled.

8. Skin Conditions

Aloe vera is very good for the skin in many ways.

- **As a moisturizer:** Applying aloe vera gel directly to the skin and then washing it out after a minute or two leaves the skin feeling soft and glowing.
- **To treat acne:** Acne is one of the most common skin problems faced today. This condition causes the appearance of painful and itchy pimples to appear on the face or shoulders. Aloe vera helps soothe the skin and tightens the pores preventing any exposure to germs. It also contains antibacterial properties and helps remove acne scars.
- **To treat sunburn:** A sunburn causes the skin to tan. Your skin becomes leathery and can sometimes be very painful too. Aloe vera helps cool the skin and helps remove the tan.
- **To treat stretch marks:** Aloe vera helps to tighten the skin and reduce the scars caused by skin stretching.
- **To treat aging of skin**: Aloe vera is used in anti-aging creams and lotions. It is a safer and more economical than surgical procedures for skin treatment.

9. Hair

Aloe is a very versatile plant. Aloe vera gel is also used as a hair care product. It helps to combat some of the most common hair problems like hair fall. Aloe vera contains a multitude of nutrients that can treat hair fall and dandruff. Using the gel regularly on the hair can make your hair smooth and shiny.

10. AIDS

The use of aloe vera plant in the treatment of AIDS is still under research and it has shown promising results. Aloe vera contains carrisyn, which appears to inhibit the growth and spread of HIV. In a study published in Journal of Advancement in Medicine, it was found that the consumption of active ingredients of an entire leaf of aloe vera on a daily basis had significantly increased their T-4 helper cell count of AIDs patients. These cells are responsible for the immunity in the body, and a patient suffering from AIDS has an immunity that is severely compromised.

Fructose – The Toxic Sugar

Sugar is an important element of our diet. There are various types of sugar derived from different sources. Some of the simple sugars, a.k.a. Monosaccharide, include glucose, fructose and galactose. The "regular" or white sugar that we use commonly in our food is sucrose, a disaccharide. Some of the other disaccharides include maltose and lactose.

Some people think of sugar as something natural, but it is entirely false. Sugar is actually manufactured from sugarcane through a series of chemical processes, so it is artificial and not a natural nutrient. Basically, sugar is 99.9% carbs and when taken in excess, can be harmful for us. It has been found that fructose has the most dangerous effects on the human system, in comparison to all other types of sugar.

Why Fructose Is Toxic for Your Health?

Earlier, like sucrose, fructose was known to be harmless but more recent scientific research has proven it to be a toxic sugar. Some of the main reasons why it is deemed harmful for human beings are:

- **Obesity & Diabetes:** High fructose intake is linked with diabetes and obesity. According to the most recent WHO reports, nearly 8.3% of the population has diabetes in America and it is expected to triple by 2050. According to the New York Times, obesity in

Americans has markedly increased in 2011. This is mainly because of the popular use of the inexpensive corn syrup, a derivative of fructose. In 2009, LA Times reported that – on an average, Americans consume about 50gms of high fructose corn syrup each day.

- **Energy Explosion:** Since fructose is the source of energy, a high intake of fructose may energize the body a bit too much. In layman's terms, eating a lot of fructose at once may become hard for your body to handle causing energy explosion in the body.
- **Heart Attack:** What happens when fructose enters your body anyway? The body excretes insulin when normal glucose sugar enters the system, but fructose is processed by the liver. The liver doesn't have enough capability to handle a lot of fructose at once and starts converting it into fat sending it into the bloodstream as body fat (triglycerides in medical terms). These triglycerides cause a risk of heart attack when produced in excess.
- **Appetite Satiation:** As the old metaphor goes – a person is never satisfied if he gets too much of something. Same is the case with fructose and the human body. When an excessive amount of fructose enters our system, it increases our craving for food even more, it will make us feel as if we're eating enough, but not really feeling satisfied.
- **Type-2 Diabetes:** Substances like high fructose from corn syrup and soft drinks are the main reasons for increasing risks of type-2 diabetes in United States. High fructose leads to reductions in insulin generation, an important element for the proper functioning of the body.
- **Gastrointestinal Problems:** Eating too much fructose can lead to gastrointestinal problems like muscle cramps, bloating and diarrhea.
- **Hypertension:** Excess fructose consumption has also been linked to hypertension and high blood pressure levels. In a 2010 study, published in the Journal of American Society of Nephrology, it was found that volunteers with an average fructose consumption of more than 74 g per day were likely to have high blood pressure. Some 4528 adults who were facing hypertension were examined

to check the relation between their fructose intake and blood pressure levels. Average daily consumption of fructose, amongst these volunteers, was found to be nearly 74 g (contained in 2.5 cans of soft drink).

- **Cancer:** Another study carried out in UCLA's Jonson Comprehensive Cancer Center showed that pancreatic tumor cells use the fructose present in the body to divide and reproduce, causing high risks for cancers.
- **Other Heart Diseases:** A research published in *Journal of Clinical Investigation* showed that overweight patients had more risks of heart and diabetes when their 25% consumed calories came from fructose-sweetened beverages in comparison to glucose sweetened beverages. 32 participants (male and female) aged 50 years were used for this study. For 10 weeks, the participants were asked to drink either glucose- or fructose-sweetened beverages which totaled up to 25% of their daily calorie intake. Obviously both type of participants gained weight, but the fructose ones gained more belly weight than the glucose ones. Belly weight has been linked to heart diseases and diabetes. Another important finding of this study was that the fructose group had developed more bad cholesterol than the sucrose group.

A lot of scientists are of the opinion that it's not just high fructose, which is dangerous for you; it is any type of excessive sugar intake in your diet that can prove harmful.

Most of us don't know what's in that can of cola, but if you are one of those who drink soda with every meal, you might have to stop and think again.

Most of the soft drinks we consume contain high amounts of fructose. In fact, drinking flavored soft drinks is the main reason why obesity is on the rise in America. Obesity is just the first step to a lot of chronic diseases like heart attacks, high cholesterol, cancer, and osteoporosis.

The choice is yours whether to control your fructose intake or keep living in ignorance.

The Best Olive Oils

There are many companies out there claiming to make the absolute best olive oils out there. They all say that *their* oil is pure, *their* oil is unprocessed, and that *their* oil is the real deal.

Obviously, you have a whole lot of various brands to choose from, so selecting one might be quite difficult, especially if you don't have much experience.

There are a few things that you will never see in high quality olive oil and I'm going to list those things for you so that you have a quick guide ready next time you go shopping.

The best olive oil will never be clear.

This is something you can look at right at the store. See, high quality olive oil will be made out of olives which have been handpicked and pressed within forty-eight hours.

The oil that gets produced this way will *never* be filtered as filtering will remove a lot of the nutrients, vitamins and lifesaving minerals you normally find in oil.

If you consume high quality olive oil, you'll lower your blood pressure, balance your cholesterol levels, decrease the risk of getting cancer as well as take advantage of antioxidants that will rejuvenate your body.

On the other hand…

The filtered (in other words clear) oil will not help much and, what's more, it will actually put you at risk of suffering from heart disease, so you need to be careful.

The best olive oil will never be diluted.

Producing high quality olive oil can be quite expensive as you need to pick olives by hand, remove leaves, stems and wash them carefully without the use of chemicals and / or machines that would damage the skin as well as the pulp.

What's more, since olive oil has been universally claimed to be extremely healthy, the demand for it is much greater than its supply.

That's why, even the best brands out there dilute olive oil by mixing it with other oils.

The solution for that is buying the best olive oils from family owned farms where you can be sure that the production process hasn't been automated and the oil hasn't been spoiled.

The best olive oil will never be exposed to light or heat.

You probably already realize that the natural light will ruin olive oil faster than anything else. That's why you'll see high quality olive oil stored in *dark bottles.*

Doing that increases the oil's shelf life and makes sure that it has all it takes to keep you and your family feeling healthy and fresh.

It's very important…

…that you understand that pretty much every brand of industrially processed olive oil is hazardous to your health.

There are toxins, chemicals and other harmful substances floating in it, so be sure to always consume the best olive oils available. You might have to pay extra for it, but believe me, it's more than worth it.

5 Hospital Secrets Every Patient Should Know

It may come to you as a surprise if we say that hospitals can make you sicker and in extreme cases, take your life. According to Consumer Reports on Health, about 100,000 deaths are linked to hospital infection every year. You never know what's going on "behind the scenes," while you lay in your ward room!

Needless to say, hospitals are run by humans and doctors can make errors too, but it becomes serious when it affects you. Isn't it?

So, what kind of mistakes do hospitals normally do? Your hospital could cause you anything from incorrect diagnosis, faulty treatment, make an entire bill for you or not give you enough care as you deserve or worse still, they could make you feel sicker than before!

Believe It or Not: Hospitals Do Make Mistakes...

In 2006, the Institute of Medicine issued a report that stated that medication mistakes is the most common medical errors that led to an estimated $3.5 billion added costs for lost wages, productivity and additional health care expenses. The report also confirmed that on an average, every day, one person per hospital gets worse due to one or the other drug error.

According to estimates by Centers for Disease Control, over 1.7 million people in a year get serious hospital-related infections. The worst part is that around 195,000 patients die each year because of hospital errors (as estimated by healthcare ratings from Health Grades).

So, it is wise to understand the dirty secrets of hospital, so you know the issues that you may encounter when you are genuinely in need of quality and timely hospital care.

Secret #1: The July Phenomena – The Month of Doom

According to the National Bureau of Economic Research, "*The average, major teaching hospital experiences an increase in risk-adjusted mortality of roughly 4 percent in the July-August period.*"

Yes, July is the worst month to land in a hospital. Why is that so? It's the month when your health will be given in the hands of new intern residents. In addition, a large number of experienced hospital personnel leave in July and are replaced by new and less experience ones. This study was carried out on 200 leading teaching hospitals by the National Bureau of Economic Research. Coincidently, 1,500 to 2,750 accelerated deaths per year happen in this span of migration.

Whether there exists an effect of July admission on intensive care mortality and length of stay in teaching hospitals or not, we can certainly say that there is no harm in delaying your surgeries till August if they're not very serious. Otherwise, who knows, you might get in hands of a resident intern who has no idea what he's dealing with!

Secret #2: Low Quality Service & Hospital Medical Errors

Hospital medical errors can cause more deaths than life threatening diseases like Diabetes, Alzheimer's, and Pneumonia. According to medical records released by Health Grades, 195,000 people each year die because of these tiny medical errors. The two main causes of these deaths are faulty diagnosis and not treating a problem in time. This means that it is possible that you may be suffering with pneumonia while the doctor diagnosis is "a viral fever"!

What is the solution to this? Well, before visiting a hospital make sure to check its ratings from U.S. Department of Health & Human Services or from independent providers such as Health Grades or The Leapfrog Group.

Secret #3: The Stranger, Anesthetist

The operating room may seem safe to you, but what if the Anesthetist isn't? Normally, people would do a background check on the surgeon but never on the Anesthetist while it is the most critical part of your surgery. A little more or less anesthesia could kill you! Although such cases are rare, they are not unheard of, and people with a previous medical condition possess even more risk in this regard.

Surgeons rarely have any idea about their anesthesiologists. And why would they? It isn't really their job, is it? So, before getting ready to go in that operating room, make sure to have a 1 to 1 discussion with the anesthesiologist.

The American Society of Anesthesiologists has done a good job in compiling some areas about which you can ask the anesthesiologist:

- His qualifications? And if he is a medical doctor trained in the field of anesthesiology.
- His previous experiences?
- Who else is going to accompany him with this anesthesia?
- Is he going to monitor the patient's heart and breathing?
- Does an anesthesiologist answer immediately when required in the recovery room?

Secret #4: Infection Payments

A lot of infections occur from hospital instruments, but that doesn't mean that the patient should pay for them. Most of the time, these infections can be prevented by proper and timely hospital care, but if not, you don't have to pay for them.

Yes, if you are a victim of any hospital error, you can say "no" and the hospital has no right to bill you.

Secret #5: Privacy and Hospital Confidentiality

Privacy is a crucial issue these days and hospital confidentiality is no reason why your surgeries won't be made public. How do you think that plastic surgery reports of Hollywood stars reach in the hands of tabloids? That's because hospitals purposely sell it to them.

Maybe you think it's not that important, but it really is, because those reports contain your identifications. In 2009, an employee of Cedars-Sinai Medical Center in Los Angeles was charged with stealing 1000 patient records and then using them for certain insurance purposes. To avoid this, check the hospital's privacy policy and request an account of all disclosures.

It is essential that we understand what we are up against when seeking hospital care. Knowledge of such hospital secrets can help a long way in getting quality and safe treatment to your problem.

The Truth about Cortisol

Cortisol, also referred to as an adrenal cortisol hormone, is perhaps the most important hormone in our body as it affects nearly all the vital organs. Cortisol falls under a class of hormones known as glucocorticoids and is secreted by the adrenal gland.

The most important job of cortisol is to help the body prepare itself and respond to stress. It also plays a key role in the following functions:

- Immune function
- Normal glucose metabolism
- Blood pressure regulation
- Inflammatory response
- Blood sugar regulation

Why cortisol carries the tag of the 'stress hormone'

There are three main reasons why cortisol is nicknamed the 'stress hormone'.

- There is an increased production of cortisol when we are in stress
- It is responsible for numerous changes in the body that occur when we are in stress
- It helps us deal with stress better

Cortisol is an integral part of our body's response to stress. A small increase in the levels of cortisol allows us to respond better to stress by:

- Providing a temporary surge in energy
- Increasing immunity temporarily
- Reducing sensitivity to pain
- Improving memory function
- Helping the body in maintaining homeostasis

Cortisol is secreted in greater amounts during the body's natural and automatic 'fight or flight' response to stress.

After the initial response to stress, marked by the increased production of cortisol and other changes in the body, it is imperative that the body's natural relaxation process is activated to allow the body to return to normal. When this does not happen, the cortisol levels in the body remain constantly high, a condition known as hypercortilism. This, in turn, can be detrimental to one's health.

Dangers of hypercortilism

Hypercortilism is linked with various health risks:

- **High blood pressure**

Cortisol increases the effects of epinephrine and norepinephrine, two hormones that increase heart rate and blood pressure. High blood pressure (medically known as hypertension), in turn, can increase the risk to various other potentially life-threatening conditions such as diabetes, heart failure, or stroke.

- **Blood sugar imbalance**

Cortisol increases the level of glucose in the blood. Hypercortilism, abnormally high levels of cortisol, in turn, leads to abnormally high glucose blood levels, a condition medically known as hyperglycemia.

- **Impaired cognitive performance**

Elevated levels of cortisol, over time, reduce and damage the number of brain cells found in the hippocampus, a major portion of the human brain that is critical to short-term memory, long-term memory, and spatial awareness.

- **Lower inflammatory responses and immunity**

Cortisol is a natural anti-inflammatory agent as it inhibits the inflammatory process. This attribute is helpful during the body's 'fight or flight' response to stress. However, the anti-inflammatory properties of cortisol become a problem when its levels are constantly high.

Cortisol lowers the levels of certain white blood cells such as lymphocytes and eosinophils, which are important for maintaining immunity, as well as a proper inflammatory response. A poor immune response, in turn, can lead to various other health conditions. Hypercortilism also leads to lower inflammatory response, which slows wound healing.

- **Cushing syndrome**

A potentially life-threatening condition, Cushing's syndrome is caused due to elevated levels of cortisol. The signs and symptoms of this health condition include: diabetes, higher-than-normal blood pressure, fatigue, moodiness, depression, pink or purple stretch marks on/around the abdomen, pronounced fatty tissue deposits on the upper back and face, new facial growth, and irregular menstrual periods in women. Cushing's syndrome is most common in people aged between 20 to 50 years, with women being five times more likely to develop the disorder than men.

- **Increased abdominal fat**

Studies conducted to understand the relation between cortisol and weight gain reveals that this hormone promotes weight gain by increasing appetite and storing fat around the abdominal area. Studies also reveal that people who have elevated levels of cortisol are likely to consume carb-rich foods, which also contributes to weight gain.

- **Clinical depression**

In normal people, the level of cortisol is highest in the morning and then reduces gradually as the day progresses. However, while the level of cortisol peaks in the morning in clinically depressed patients, it does not reduce in the afternoon or evening.

Although the exact role that cortisol plays in promoting depression has not been established, it is largely believed that cortisol contributes to depression by reducing the levels of serotonin, a hormone that promotes a feeling of well-being.

Tips to prevent hypercortilism

Chronic stress is listed as one of the most prominent cause of hypercortilism. You can reduce your risk of hypercortilism by learning and practicing stress management techniques such as:

- Meditation
- Yoga
- Breathing exercises
- Self-hypnosis
- Guided imagery
- Exercise
- Listening to music

Infrared Sauna Benefits

Hundreds, even thousands of years ago, people turned to heat therapy as a source of healing. Sauna is one of the best ways to immediately sooth achy muscles and relax busy minds. Health professionals worldwide recognize the benefits of saunas to promote blood circulation and oxygenation of body tissues, relief aches, pains, and general stiffness; eliminate body toxins by promoting perspiration; and even to help burn some unwanted calories.

Unlike traditional saunas that can be uncomfortably hot, far-infrared sauna uses light to create heat. They are a great alternative to the traditional sauna, especially for elderly and people with asthma, as it warms objects without warming the air between it and the object. It allows you to sweat without feeling the intense heat of a regular sauna.

What Is Far-Infrared?

Far-infrared heat is a safe form of naturally occurring energy. Infrared rays have a longer wavelength and cannot be seen by a human eye. Our bodies are able to absorb these rays when in direct contact. This heat doesn't raise the temperature of the air but goes 2-3" into the body heats the body directly, thus providing all the benefits of natural sunlight without the harmful effects of ultraviolet radiation.

Infrared saunas gained a lot popularity due to its many health benefits. They are available in all shapes, sizes and prices from full size cabins that can seat up to 4 people to the small individual and portable sauna bags, whatever your needs there will be something for you.

Health Benefits of Infrared Sauna

- The infrared rays enter the body and converts into energy which stimulates the body tissues. This helps body to change fat cells into sweat and resultantly a person loses fat and weight. You can burn 400-600 calories in just one 30-minute session.
- Helps flush out toxins.
- Improves metabolism.
- Relaxes muscles and helps eliminate shoulder, neck, and back pain.
- Speeds up healing process. People who suffer from sprains and strains must use sauna to recover quickly.
- Improves blood circulation.
- Relieves arthritis pain.
- Boosts immune system.
- Helps relax and rejuvenate the body.
- Removes oil, dirt, makeup from clogged pores and improves skin problems like acne, rashes and scars.

Precautions

- No alcohol usage prior to a sauna session.
- Drink plenty of water before and after sauna.
- Children must be accompanied and they should take a bath under supervision.
- If you have some medical problem or pregnant, consult your doctor before using sauna.

Recommended session time is about 10-15 minutes. You can extend it to about 20 minutes. Just remember that excess is never a good thing. Always do your own research and be aware of the benefits and limitations of an infrared sauna. Never check your physical limits while using it and it is always better to first learn how to use it and what would the best method for you. The limitations of sauna differ for each one of us and similarly the benefits also differ and depend upon the health condition of the person. Remember, always respect your body limitations.

10 Life-Saving Blood Tests

If you want to know your heart attack risk, you get your cholesterol checked, right? Wrong! Cholesterol tests fail to identify almost half of people at risk for having a heart attack, stroke or other potentially deadly cardiovascular issues.

With cardiovascular disease as the number one cause of death in the United States, causing an astonishing 2,200 deaths every day, doctors include a cholesterol test as part of every checkup. Unfortunately, relying on total cholesterol, LDL and HDL levels is often not enough to accurately assess your cardiovascular health.

Fortunately, there are newer, more effective tests that can better predict your cardiovascular risk. These 10 lifesaving blood tests include:

- **C-reactive protein (CRP)** – protein produced by the liver increases during whole-body inflammation. In the long term such inflammation can damage healthy tissue and lead to heart disease.
- **Homocysteine** - amino acid that is thought to damage the cells that line your arteries.
- **Triglycerides** – a form of fat made in the body that is a risk factor for cardiovascular disease.
- **Apolipoprotein B (Apo B)** - major protein found in cholesterol particles, forming the majority of the LDL cholesterol particles.

- **Lipoprotein(a)** – made up of LDL cholesterol particles attached to a protein called apo(a), which inflames the blood and makes it more prone to clotting.
- **Very Low-Density Lipoprotein (VLDL)** – contains highest triglyceride levels and helps cholesterol build up on the walls of arteries.
- **LDL size** – LDL particles range in size from large and buoyant to small and dense, which easily invades the artery wall and begins the process of atherosclerosis.
- **Hemoglobin A1C** – shows your average blood sugar levels over the past 2 to 3 months and correlates well with your heart disease risk.
- **Fibrinogen** – protein found in the blood that makes it sticky and helps it clot; having too much fibrinogen can cause a clot to form in an artery, leading to a heart attack or stroke.
- **Cardiac troponin** – indicates that damage has been done to the heart.

You can get more information about these tests and other blood panels that can be used to help diagnosis potentially serious conditions, as well as improve your overall health, through the Blood Test Results Decoded program. This program was designed to help you understand what your blood tests are telling you so you can start a conversation with your doctor about optimizing your health instead of blindly guessing at what's wrong and what diet, vitamins, minerals and other supplements could help prevent potential disease and help you feel better, more energetic and more like the you that you always knew you should be.

Phosphatidylserine for Brain Nutrition

Phosphatidylserine belongs to a class of chemicals known as phospholipids, which are fat-soluble chemicals that are vital for cell membranes.

Phosphatidylserine is a non-essential nutrient. The term 'non-essential nutrient' refers to nutrients that our body can produce naturally. We can also procure Phosphatidylserine from food. With that said, it is important to note that a typical diet usually contains only a small amount of Phosphatidylserine.

Although Phosphatidylserine deficiency is not a serious issue since our body can naturally produce this chemical, elderly people, especially those who experience symptoms of age-related cognitive decline, are less likely to synthesize adequate amounts of Phosphatidylserine. Such individuals are also more likely to benefit from Phosphatidylserine supplements.

Apart from elderly people with age-related memory impairment and other cognitive decline, those who are at increased risk of anxiety, depression, and other mental disorders also stand to gain from Phosphatidylserine supplements. These supplements are also apt for athletes and individuals who work out intensely.

Bovine-derived Phosphatidylserine vs. Soy-based Phosphatidylserine

Until recently, almost all Phosphatidylserine supplements were bovine-derived. However, this is no longer the case now. Many commercial Phosphatidylserine supplements sold today are soy-based. The main reason for this 'switch' was the possibility of infections such as mad cow disease. With that said, it is important to note that a single case of an animal disease occurring due to bovine-based Phosphatidylserine supplements has been recorded.

Soy-based Phosphatidylserine, preliminary animal researches declare, have the same positive effects on the human brain as animal-derived Phosphatidylserine.

What are the benefits of Phosphatidylserine?

Phosphatidylserine is believed to:

- Improve memory
- Boost learning
- Increase attention and vigilance
- Enhance mental acuity
- Improve concentration
- Improve mood
- Relieve or reduce the intensity of depression
- Reduce stress
- Inhibit increase in cortisol due to exercise and stress

The more important benefits of Phosphatidylserine are given below in detail:

Phosphatidylserine and Alzheimer's Disease

Phosphatidylserine is known to reduce symptoms of Alzheimer's disease, a degenerative mental disorder. Several studies conducted so far have revealed that Phosphatidylserine supplements are most effective in individuals who predominantly exhibit less severe symptoms associated with this condition.

Phosphatidylserine and Senile Dementia

Phosphatidylserine reduces symptoms of senile dementia and age-related memory impairment. This chemical, studies show, can improve language skills, memory, and attention in aging individuals with deteriorating thinking skills.

Phosphatidylserine and Depression

Phosphatidylserine can stimulate neurotransmitters and brain chemicals that regulate mood. For instance, this chemical can lead to an increase in the production of dopamine, a neurotransmitter that plays a key role in regulating mood and emotions. Dopamine improves mood and increases positive thoughts and feelings. Individuals who are depressed or are suffering from anxiety typically have low levels of dopamine.

The fact that an increase in dopamine production can reduce depression and anxiety is the main reason why health experts reckon that Phosphatidylserine, which stimulates the production of Dopamine, can be helpful in the treatment of depression and anxiety. You must always consult your doctor before using Phosphatidylserine for treating anxiety, depression, or any other mental disorder.

Phosphatidylserine and Muscle Recovery

A study which appeared in *Journal of the International Society of Sports Nutrition* stated that phospholipids can boost the capacity to exercise and may also speed up muscle recovery after an intense workout.

The study found that Phosphatidylserine improved exercise capacity of individuals during high-intensity running and cycling. This study also suggested that phospholipids, such as Phosphatidylserine, may enhance performance during exercise. In addition, this chemical has a stimulatory effect on certain hormones, including cortisol, leading to a reduced perception of soreness in muscles following an intense workout.

Phosphatidylserine and Attention Deficit Hyperactive Disorder (ADHD)

Studies show that this phospholipid can reduce certain symptoms of ADHD such as nervousness, anxiety, and hyperactivity. Phosphatidylserine achieves by improving brain circulation.

Phosphatidylserine, without a doubt, offers numerous benefits. However, the use of Phosphatidylserine may not be recommended in certain conditions, or you may need to observe certain precautions.

AlphaBRAIN™ supplement contain Phosphadylserine and helps increase focus and mental clarity to help achieve improved cognitive functioning. It provides a strong foundation to enhance the body's endogenous production and maintenance of key neurotransmitters.

Phosphatidylserine and Pregnancy

This non-essential nutrient should not be used by a pregnant woman unless her doctor recommends it. This is because the safety of Phosphatidylserine supplements in pregnant women has not been adequately studied.

Phosphatidylserine and Breastfeeding

Breastfeeding women should consult their doctor before using Phosphatidylserine supplements. The safety of Phosphatidylserine supplements in such women has not been adequately examined.

Phosphatidylserine and Drug Interactions

If you are taking certain drugs such as anticholinergic medications, cholinergic drugs, and acetylcholinesterase inhibiting drugs, you must consult your physician before using Phosphatidylserine. These medications and several others may interfere with Phosphatidylserine function and/or vice-versa.

What is the correct dosage of Phosphatidylserine?

It is recommended that you use Phosphatidylserine exactly as recommended in the instructions on the label or as directed by your doctor. For senile dementia, other age-related cognitive decline, and Alzheimer's disease, the recommended daily dosage is 300 mg, administered in three small dosages of 100 mg each.

Are there any side effects of Phosphatidylserine?

Phosphatidylserine is not known to cause any side effects as long as the recommended dosage of 300 mg is adhered to. However, if you take more than 300 mg of Phosphatidylserine daily, you may experience side effects such as upset stomach and insomnia.

Improve Metabolism with Digestive Enzymes

The human body is an incredibly complex network of systems where each function is interrelated to the other by signaling components. The development and maintenance of all these systems is based on intricate and precise working conditions of biological catalysts called enzymes. All human bodies are capable of producing all the enzymes they require that are vital to the smooth running of the splendid show called life.

What are enzymes?

Every simple or complex process in our body is possible because of a series of chemical reactions. These reactions are governed by enzymes which either hasten the speed of the reaction by exponential rates or make otherwise impossible reactions take place in its presence. Essentially all enzymes are made up of proteins. What is amazing about these enzymes is that even though they participate in a reaction, they remain unaltered in terms of their chemical composition while they convert biological reactants (substrates) into the required products. Because of this property, they can be reused multiple times, depending on the requirement of the product.

What are the main properties of enzymes?

As we have established, enzymes are proteins that take part in a reaction without changing their own chemical properties. Besides this, it is important to understand other properties of enzymes.

- **Enzymes are highly specific:** An enzyme is not only function specific but substrate specific.
- **Enzyme catalysed reactions are reversible:** They can catalyse the both the forward reactions (substrate to product) and backward reactions (product to substrate)
- **Enzymes are reactive:** As proteins, enzymes have a temperature and pH at which they denature and lose their activity. In most cases, denaturation is an irreversible process. The functionality or the activity' of the enzyme is greatly affected by the prevalent temperatures and pH of the reaction. Therefore, every enzyme has an optimum temperature and pH at which the activity of the enzyme is the highest. Consequently, minimum activity is also evident at a particular point of these parameters.

What are digestive enzymes?

As the name suggests, these are a set of enzymes that aid smooth digestion of food. These enzymes are strategically secreted and present in various parts of the alimentary canal. The food we eat is systematically broken down from complex to gradually simpler compounds before they are absorbed and then distributed throughout the body. Digestive enzymes are present in the mouth, stomach, pancreas and the small intestine.

There are 4 categories of digestive enzymes:

- **Proteolytic enzymes:** Catalyse the breakdown of proteins to amino acids.
- **Lipolytic enzymes:** Catalyse the breakdown of fatty acids and glycerol.

- **Amylolytic enzymes:** Catalyse the breakdown starch to simple sugars.
- **Nucleolytic enzymes:** Catalyse the breakdown of nucleic acids.

What are digestive enzyme supplements?

The digestive enzymes especially in the stomach take some time to get secreted and act on the food. Besides this, our growing sedentary life-style causes the food to remain undigested for longer than required. Digestive enzyme supplements help speed up digestion. Consuming these supplements before or after a heavy meal can be very helpful.

What kind of digestive enzyme supplements are good for us?

There are several types of digestive enzymes. However, there are some digestive enzymes that play a more obvious role in the process. Supplements are taken to break down different kinds of food. The supplement that one chooses should contain the following essential enzymes.

- **Papain:** It is derived from papaya and extremely effective in digesting proteins and tenderizing meat.
- **Amylase:** This enzyme breaks starch into its component sugars namely glucose.
- **Lipase:** This enzyme breaks down long chain fatty acids and consequently digesting fats.
- **Lactase:** This works to break down dairy products.
- **Bromelain:** This is an enzyme which is found in pineapple. It is a remarkable enzyme capable of digesting protein.

What are the main benefits of digestive enzymes?

Now, the question lingers as to why digestive enzyme supplements should even be considered taking, since our body produces all the enzymes required. One must understand that the more enzymes that the body uses for digestion is proportional to the exhaustion of the same. Therefore, in order to have a constant supply of one's naturally secreted digestive enzymes to maintain a longer and healthier living, one must take these supplements.

- The most obvious benefit is the decrease in indigestion and bloated feeling of the stomach, since lesser acid is produced in the body for digestion.
- Reduction in the number of ulcers.
- Relief from hiatal hernias.
- Reduced food allergies.

Digestive Enzymes – Do try this at home!

To test how good your supplement is, there is a very simple experiment that you can conduct. Take two bowls of thick oatmeal. Leave one of the bowls as is and add the prescribed amount of digestive enzyme supplement in the other. After about half an hour, the oatmeal in the latter should start to look less thick and almost watery.

This shows that the oatmeal was partially digested which saves the body much energy in digestion and nutrients are absorbed much faster.

Importance of Electrolytes

Electrolytes are important elements and compounds needed by our body cells. Chemically, electrolytes are substances that become ions in solution and acquire the capacity to conduct electricity. In a balanced amount, they help maintain the numerous functions of the millions of cells in the human body. Without these electrolytes, our muscles won't be able to move, our nerves will have trouble sending communication to and from the brain, and the rest of bodily functions can become so dysregulated that it makes possible for vital organs to shut down.

What is an electrolyte?

Electrolyte is a medical term for ions. Ions, as you may know, are of the following two types:

- Positively-charged
- Negatively-charged

Positively-charged ions move toward the cathode, while negatively-charged ions move towards the anode. An electrolyte, in simplest terms, is used for defining any substance that contains free ions to conduct electricity.

The human body and electrolytes

We cannot exist without electrolytes. In fact, no higher form of life can survive without them.

Our body fluids such as blood, interstitial fluid or tissue fluid (solution that surrounds our cells), and plasma contain electrolytes. These body fluids contain the following electrolytes:

- Sodium (Na^+)
- Calcium (Ca^{2+})
- Potassium (K^+)
- Magnesium (Mg^{2+})
- Bicarbonate (HCO_3^-)
- Chloride (Cl^-)
- Hydrogen carbonate (HCO_3^-)
- Hydrogen phosphate (HPO_4^{2-})

Electrolytes regulate important body functions such as:

- Nerve and muscle function
- Dehydration
- Rebuilding of tissues that are damaged
- Blood pressure
- Blood pH levels

To contract, our muscles require sodium, calcium, and potassium. In case the levels of these are below normal, our muscles become too weak. Similarly, if the levels are above normal, muscle contractions can be too severe.

The other important function electrolytes have is to regulate muscle and nerve function. Our nerve cells and muscle cells require electrolytes for maintaining voltage across the cell membranes. This allows the cells to transport electrical impulses to other cells.

Regulation of electrolytes in the human body

The human body needs to maintain the levels of electrolytes. The kidney and other hormones play a vital role in regulating electrolyte levels.

Symptoms of electrolyte imbalance

The most common type of electrolyte imbalance is hyperkalemia (too much potassium), hypokalemia (too little potassium), hypernatremia (too much sodium), hyponatremia (too little sodium), hypercalcemia (too much calcium), and hypocalcemia (too little calcium).

The symptoms of electrolyte imbalance depend on the electrolyte that is out of balance. For instance, symptoms of hypercalcemia may be different from those of hypernatremia. That said, in case of electrolyte imbalance, you will experience one or more of the below-mentioned symptoms:

- Twitching
- Muscle weakness and/or general weakness
- Confusion
- Numbness
- Seizures
- Fatigue
- Convulsions
- Muscle spasm
- Fast or slow heartbeat
- Changes in blood pressure

What causes electrolyte imbalance

One of the most common cause electrolyte depletion, particularly potassium and sodium, is excessive sweating. When you sweat profusely, for instance during and after exercise, the body loses electrolytes through sweat. That is why people who play sports or exercises regularly need to drink fluids, such as sports drinks, which contain electrolytes. However, excessive use of sports drinks is not recommended because they usually contain sugar and artificial flavors that may be harmful.

If you regularly play sports or exercise, you must either consume electrolyte-enriched drinks that do not contain sugar, such as Alacer Electro Mix Natural, or consume electrolyte-rich foods, such as apples, oranges, or tomatoes, in larger quantities.

Chronic diarrhea or vomiting can also lead to electrolyte imbalance. To prevent seizures and dehydration that can occur due to loss of electrolytes, you must replenish them quickly. For this, you will need to drink fluids that contain electrolytes.

In addition to the above, other situations in which electrolyte imbalance may occur include the following:

- Kidney disorder
- Cancer treatment
- Use of certain drugs like ACE inhibitors or diuretics
- Heart failure
- Bulimia

Electrolyte imbalance and gerontology

Elderly people are more vulnerable to electrolyte imbalance. The primary reason for this is poor kidney function. As we age, our kidneys do not work as well as they used to do in our younger years. This is why elderly people must take proper precautions to prevent electrolyte imbalance. To prevent electrolyte imbalance, it is essential that you keep yourself properly hydrated all the time.

Foods that are rich in electrolytes

While there are many drinks available that replenish electrolytes, the best way of maintaining optimal electrolyte level is by eating foods that are rich in electrolytes.

Here are the names of foods that you can eat to maintain electrolyte balance in the body:

- **Fruits –** Most fruits are rich in electrolytes. These include apples, peaches, oranges, melons, and bananas.
- **Vegetables –** Besides offering antioxidants and other nutrients, vegetables, in general, are rich in electrolytes. These include spinach, squash, collard greens, kale, mustard greens, broccoli, peas, red onions, sweet potatoes, baked potatoes, and Brussels sprouts.
- **Beans –** Mung, red, lima, pinto and white beans are an excellent source of mineral-rich electrolytes.
- **Whole grains** - Whole grains are particularly rich in electrolytes such as magnesium and calcium.
- **Meat and seafood –** Pork, sardines, and beef are rich in chloride. Chicken contains high amounts of calcium as soon as they are organic.

To summarize, electrolytes are essential for maintaining numerous bodily functions, and their deficiency and excess can cause various health issues. The best way to keep electrolyte balance in check is by through sugar-free, electrolyte-rich drinks or natural foods.

Egg-Zackly

Eggs have long been touted as a cholesterol enhancer. You were led to believe for years that eggs are not good for only in moderation. Well let's dispel this old wives tail once and for all.

Eggs can be high in the pro-inflammatory omega-6 fatty acid arachidonic acid, partly because chickens are fed soy and corn rather than their natural diet. One large conventional egg, to be exact, contains an imbalance of 574 mg of omega-6s and 37 mg of omega-3 fatty acids.

1 egg packs about 7 grams of very high-quality protein. While their saturated fat sometimes gets an undeserved bad rep, eggs actually provide a balance of saturated, monounsaturated, and polyunsaturated fats.

Yes, the fat is all in the yolk; so are the nutrients. Among its array of nutrients, the United States Department of Agriculture (USDA) reports 1 egg yolk provides:

- 245 IUs of vitamin A
- 37 IUs of vitamin D
- 19 mg potassium
- 25 mcg folate
- 22 mg calcium

According to Dr. Jonny Bowden in his book *The 150 Healthiest Foods on Earth,* one large egg yolk also provides 300 mcg of choline, which forms betaine to help lower homocysteine (a risk factor for heart disease). Choline also helps make phosphatidylcholine to benefit your liver, nervous system, and brain.

Experts have come out against the rampant anti-cholesterol mania. We now know that dietary cholesterol has almost no impact on blood cholesterol, but some people still fear this crucial molecule that helps make your sex hormones and vitamin D.

Many people think of cholesterol as being harmful, but the truth is that it's essential for your body to function.

Cholesterol contributes to the membrane structure of every single cell in your body.

Your body also needs it to make hormones and vitamin D, and perform various other important functions. Simply put, you could not survive without it.

When people talk about cholesterol in relation to heart health, they usually aren't talking about cholesterol itself.

They are actually referring to the structures that carry cholesterol in the bloodstream. These are called lipoproteins.

Lipoproteins are made of fat (lipid) on the inside and protein on the outside.

There are several kinds of lipoproteins, but the two most relevant to heart health are low-density lipoprotein (LDL) and high-density lipoprotein (HDL).

Taking it a step further and looking at LDL particle size and inflammatory markers like HS-CRP and A1C levels are more of true indicator if you are at risk for heart disease, not the overall number of total cholesterol.

The smaller more abundant particles sizes you have the greater the risk, the larger the particle size the risk is less. Why you may ask? This is because the general increase in LDL particles typically reflects an increase in large LDL particles, not small, dense LDL. People who have mainly large LDL particles actually have a lower risk of heart disease because the larger sizes flow freely and do not create plaque.

Measurements of lipids levels in blood are frequently used to assess the risk of future heart disease. The most commonly used measurements are total cholesterol, triglycerides and HDL-C. These numbers are then used to calculate LDL-C, which has been found to be strongly correlated with the risk of heart disease.

Recently measurements of atherogenic lipoprotein particles, such as LDL-P (LDL particle number), apolipoprotein-B (apoB) and lipoprotein-a have been found to be very useful to assess risk.

LDL-P measures the actual number of LDL particles (particle concentration). LDL-P may be a stronger predictor of cardiovascular events than LDL-C. Low LDL-P is a much stronger predictor of low risk than low LDL-C. In fact, about 30 – 40% of those with low LDL-C may have elevated LDL-P. Therefore you can have low LDL-C but still be at risk for heart disease, particularly if your LDL-P is elevated. Discordance is considered present if LDL-C differs from LDL-P.

LDL-C is a measure of the cholesterol mass within LDL-particles. LDL-C only indirectly reflects the atherogenic potential of LDL particles. ApoB and LDL-P on the other hand reflect the number of atherogenic particles, with no mention of cholesterol mass. ApoB and LDL-P are believed to be better risk predictors than LDL-C.

I can't tell you the amount of clients that have come to me that have been on statins for years and think they are doing great because their total cholesterol number went from 250 to 150. The problem here is, the doctor never did a particle size cholesterol test to show the ratios. More often than not I have seen that total number go down in these clients but their small particle size numbers (the really bad ones) remain high or even GO UP!! This puts them into a false sende of security until crisis hits.

Many recent studies have looked into the importance of LDL-particle size. Studies show that people whose LDL particles are predominantly small and dense, have a threefold greater risk of coronary heart disease. Furthermore, the large and fluffy type of LDL may be protective.

Not All Eggs are Created Equal

Getting back to the wonderful egg and the problem we have today is that there are several varieties of eggs available in stores today.

- **Brown or white eggs**
- **Sizes like jumbo, large, medium, small, peewee**

- **Standard cage eggs, cage-free, free-range, organic, and specialty type eggs like omega-three fatty acid and other nutrient-added eggs**

So how do you choose?

Free range - this term is essentially meaningless. Government only loosely regulates the definition of "free range," and egg producers have jumped at the opportunity to print some new labels and charge more money in return for giving their hens occasional access to a tiny patch of dirt. According to the Department of Agriculture, egg "producers must demonstrate to the Agency that the poultry has been allowed access to the Outside" In other words, there needs to be a door to the chicken cage, and it needs to be open part of the time, but the chickens can still eat substandard food and live in cramped conditions.

Cage Free - Even more meaningless than "free range," this term has no legal definition. Technically, cage free hens don't live in stifling metal cages; instead, they might still live in hot, smelly, overcrowded henhouses! Some cage free hens' lives aren't much qualitatively better than those who live in cages and most still aren't getting any access to the outdoors, but they're generally raised with better food and better treatment.

Organic - Organic is more useful and easy to pin down. Organic egg producing hens are given organic feed, no antibiotics (unless in the case of an outbreak), and limited access to the outdoors (just a door to their cage or barn, really). These are better than your average mass-produced egg, but your best bet is still to find a truly pasture-raised egg.

All Natural - This is the most useless, all-encompassing term for anything. All produce is natural. These eggs weren't created in a lab by a team of white coats. Even the most steroid-pumped, antibiotic-immersed hens produce "natural" eggs the way nature intended: by laying them.

Omega 3 fortified - Omega-3 fortified eggs come from hens fed flax, linseed, or a direct supplement. Omega-3 fortified eggs also tend to come from organic, cage-free birds, so they're generally better.

Now the only time I have found eggs to be bad for my clients is when they test high for arachidonic acid on a Micronutrient test. More often than not it's because they are eating low quality eggs from chickens that are eating a menu of GMO corn and feed. If my clients test high on this scale then I get them off of eggs for a few weeks then gradually re-introduce them back into their menu but only the organic kind.

Study's Data Show Egg Consumption Actually Promotes Health

Another interesting analysis has been made by another author Ned Kock, who specializes in nonlinear variance-based structural equation modeling. Using a model to test for the "moderating effect," he demonstrates how the egg consumption data from the featured study actually shows that egg consumption promotes health.

By looking into the effect that the number of eggs consumed per week had on the association between LDL cholesterol and plaque formation, the data shows that the highest amount of plaque is associated with the lowest LDL cholesterol levels... This is interesting, to say the least, since egg yolks are "supposed to" raise your LDL (bad) cholesterol levels thereby causing plaque buildup.

For example, previous studies from the Harvard School of Health found that consumption of more than 6 eggs per week does not increase the risk of stroke.

Eating two eggs a day does not adversely affect endo-thel-ial function (an aggregate measure of cardiac risk) in healthy adults, supporting the view that dietary cholesterol may be less detrimental to cardiovascular health than previously thought

Proteins in cooked eggs are converted by gastrointestinal enzymes, producing peptides that act as ACE inhibitors (common prescription medications for lowering blood pressure)

Ideally, the yolks should be consumed raw as the heat will damage many of the highly perishable nutrients in the yolk. Additionally, the cholesterol in the yolk can be oxidized with high temperatures, especially when it is in contact with the iron present in the whites and cooked, as in scrambled eggs, and such oxidation contributes to chronic inflammation in your body, which is definitely associated with increased risk of plaque formation and heart disease.

However, if you're eating raw eggs, they MUST be organic pastured eggs. You do not want to consume conventionally-raised eggs raw, as they're much more likely to be contaminated with pathogens such as salmonella. Organic pastured eggs are also far superior when it comes to nutrient content. In a 2007 egg-testing project, Mother Earth News compared the official U.S. Department of Agriculture (USDA) nutrient data for commercial eggs with eggs from hens raised on pasture and found that the latter typically contains:

1/3 less cholesterol 2/3 more vitamin A

3 times more vitamin E

1/4 less saturated fat 2 times more omega-3 fatty acids 7 times more beta-carotene

The dramatically superior nutrient levels are most likely the result of the differences in diet between free ranging, pastured hens and commercially-farmed hens. An egg is considered organic if the chicken was only fed organic food, which means it will not have accumulated high levels of pesticides from the grains (mostly GM corn) fed to typical chickens. It's important to realize that an egg can be organic without being pasture-raised. "Pastured" means the chickens have been allowed to forage for its natural food sources outside, and is your best guarantee of a high quality egg. A deep yellow or orange yolk is a telltale sign of high-quality organic pastured eggs.

How to Find Fresh Pastured Organic Eggs

The key to getting high quality eggs is to buy them locally, either from an organic farm or farmers market. Fortunately, finding organic eggs locally is far easier than finding raw milk as virtually every rural area has individuals with chickens. Farmers markets are a great way to meet the people who produce your food. With face-to-face contact, you can get your questions answered and know exactly what you're buying. Better yet, visit the farm and ask for a tour. To locate a free-range pasture farm, try asking your local health food store, or check out the following web listings:

Local Harvest
USDA's farmer's market listing
Eat Wild

If you absolutely must purchase your eggs from a commercial grocery store, look for ones that are marked free-range organic. They're like still going to originate from a mass-production facility (so you'll want to be careful about eating them raw), but it's about as good as it gets if you can't find a local source.

I would strongly encourage you to AVOID ALL omega-3 eggs, as they are some of the least healthy for you. These eggs typically come from chickens that are fed poor-quality sources of omega-3 fats that are already oxidized. Also, omega-3 eggs perish much faster than non-omega-3 eggs.

https://www.hsph.harvard.edu/nutritionsource/food-features/eggs/

8 Ingredients You Never Want to See on Your Nutrition Label

The Food and Drug Administration has approved more than 3,000 food additives, most of which you've never heard of. But the truth is, you don't have to know them all. You just need to be able to parse out the bad stuff. Do that and you'll have a pretty good idea how your future will shape up—whether you'll end up overweight and unhealthy or turn out to be fit, happy, and energized.

BHA

This preservative is used to prevent rancidity in foods that contain oils. Unfortunately, BHA (butylated hydroxyanisole) has been shown to cause cancer in rats, mice, and hamsters. The reason the FDA hasn't banned it is largely technical—the cancers all occurred in the rodents' fore-stomachs, an organ that humans don't have. Nevertheless, the study, published in the *Japanese Journal of Cancer Research*, concluded that BHA was "reasonably anticipated to be a carcinogen," and as far as I'm concerned, that's reason enough to eliminate it from your diet.

Parabens

These synthetic preservatives are used to inhibit mold and yeast in food. The problem is parabens may also disrupt your body's hormonal balance. A study in *Food Chemical Toxicology* found that daily ingestion decreased sperm and testosterone production in rats, and parabens have been found present in breast cancer tissues.

Partially Hydrogenated Oil

I've harped on this before, but it bears repeating: Don't confuse "0 g trans-fat" with being trans-fat-free. The FDA allows products to claim zero grams of trans fat as long as they have less than half a gram per serving. That means they can have 0.49 grams per serving and still be labeled a no-trans-fat food. Considering that two grams is the absolute most you ought to consume in a day, those fractions can quickly add up. The telltale sign that your snack is soiled with the stuff? Look for partially hydrogenated oil on the ingredient statement. If it's anywhere on there, then you're ingesting artery-clogging trans-fat.

Sodium Nitrite

Nitrites and nitrates are used to inhibit botulism-causing bacteria and to maintain processed meats' pink hues, which is why the FDA allows their use. Unfortunately, once ingested, nitrite can fuse with amino acids (of which meat is a prime source) to form nitrosamines, powerful carcinogenic compounds. Ascorbic and eryth-orbic acids—essentially vitamin C—have been shown to decrease the risk, and most manufacturers now add one or both to their products, which has helped. Still, the best way to reduce risk is to limit your intake.

Caramel Coloring

This additive wouldn't be dangerous if you made it the old-fashioned way—with water and sugar, on top of a stove. But the food industry follows a different recipe: They treat sugar with ammonia, which can produce some nasty carcinogens. How carcinogenic are these compounds? A Center for Science in the Public Interest report asserted that the high levels of caramel color found in soda account for roughly 15,000 cancers in the U.S. annually. Another good reason to scrap soft drinks?

Casto-reum

Castoreum is one of the many nebulous "natural ingredients" used to flavor food. Though it isn't harmful, it is unsettling. Castoreum is a substance made from beavers' castor sacs, or anal scent glands. These glands produce potent secretions that help the animals mark their territory in the wild. In the food industry, however, 1,000 pounds of the unsavory ingredient are used annually to imbue foods—usually vanilla or raspberry flavored—with a distinctive, musky flavor.

You'll find it in: Potentially any food containing "natural ingredients"

Food Dyes

Plenty of fruit-flavored candies and sugary cereals don't contain a single gram of produce, but instead rely on artificial dyes and flavorings to suggest a relationship with nature. Not only do these dyes allow manufacturers to mask the drab colors of heavily processed foods, but certain hues have been linked to more serious ailments. A *Journal of Pediatrics* study linked Yellow 5 to hyperactivity in children, Canadian researchers found Yellow 6 and Red 40 to be contaminated with known carcinogens, and Red 3 is known to cause tumors. The bottom line? Avoid artificial dyes as much as possible.

Hydrolyzed Vegetable Protein

Hydrolyzed vegetable protein, used as a flavor enhancer, is plant protein that has been chemically broken down into amino acids. One of these acids, glutamic acid, can release free glutamate. When this glutamate joins with free sodium in your body, they form monosodium glutamate (MSG), an additive known to cause adverse reactions—headaches, nausea, and weakness, among others—in sensitive individuals. When MSG is added to products directly, the FDA requires manufacturers to disclose its inclusion on the ingredient statement. But when it occurs as a byproduct of hydrolyzed protein, the FDA allows it to go unrecognized.

Are Air Freshers Bad for Your Health?

The air freshener is largely considered to be a safe and useful household product. The 'useful' part still holds true, but doubts are being raised about its safety. Recent studies reveal that various health hazards may be lurking behind the sweet scent of air fresheners. Are these warnings real? Read on to know more about the potential health dangers of air fresheners.

The warning bells were first sounded when the findings of a study done by the Natural Resources Defense Council (NRDC) were made public. NRDC tested 14 random air fresheners and found that 12 of them contained phthalates, chemicals that are extremely dangerous to humans.

Other studies have also concluded that air fresheners may be potentially dangerous. Before we look further into the various other possible health risks associated with air fresheners, besides the ones phthalates is known to cause, it is imperative that we understand the health consequences of exposure to phthalates – the substance at the center of controversy surrounding air fresheners.

Numerous studies have linked phthalates with poor semen quality, abnormalities in genital development, and changes in reproductive hormone levels. Certain types of phthalates are known to cause serious reproductive harm or birth defects. In addition, exposure to phthalates can cause and/or precipitate asthma and allergic symptoms.

All in all, the verdict is unanimous – that exposure to phthalates in high quantities can have serious health consequences.

What we know is that exposure to phthalates in high concentration is dangerous and many, if not most, air fresheners contain phthalates. The concentration of phthalates in air fresheners is not known to us. We also do not know at what concentration phthalates become dangerous.

The government regulatory bodies in the USA do not make it mandatory for manufacturers of air fresheners to list phthalates content on their product labels. The initiative, health experts argue, must come from the regulatory bodies. They should conduct studies on phthalates present in air fresheners to establish at what concentration this substance becomes harmful. Also, it should be mandatory for the manufacturers to list phthalates content on their products. As of now, there is no way of telling which air freshener contains phthalates and which one doesn't.

So, what should customers do in such a scenario? Should they stop using air fresheners and look for other healthy alternatives to keep their homes smelling fresh? It may well be prudent to use natural alternatives to keep the air in your home odor free – at least until the regulatory bodies make it mandatory to list phthalates content on all products that contain this substance.

Exposure to phthalates is not the only danger of using air fresheners. Various other studies have shown that many of them also contain other harmful chemicals called volatile organic compounds (VOCs for short). Let's take a look at two such studies:

A study presented at the yearly meeting of ACAAI (American College of Allergy, Asthma, and Immunology) revealed that air fresheners usually contain VOCs such as limonene, formaldehyde, and petroleum distillates. VOCs can cause and/or precipitate asthma and other allergic reactions. The study also revealed that 34% of asthmatics experienced health problems after they were exposed to air fresheners.

A study conducted by the European Consumers Union in 2005 also found VOCs such as formaldehyde, limonene, and benzene in air fresheners. VOCs are not only linked to asthma, irritation of the respiratory tract, dizziness, and headaches, but to certain types of cancers as well. For instance, benzene is linked with leukemia, and formaldehyde is known to cause upper respiratory tract cancer.

According to experts, 'unscented' and 'all-natural' air fresheners may also not be safe. This apprehension is based on the fact a few of the 14 air fresheners the NRDC tested were labeled as 'unscented' or 'all-natural'.

There are few organic air fresheners on the market. Always do your research to ensure you are not putting yours and your family health in danger.

A Fruit That Cures the Flu

As winter approaches, there's tons of talk about this year's looming flu season. Actually, it's a lot more like yelling… and it goes something like, "Get your flu shot NOW!"

But in spite of this, you might still end up catching the flu. And that's where a study I'm going to share with you today can make a huge difference. It's about a natural fruit extract with the amazing ability to help you get rid of the flu just as effectively as Tamiflu – a commonly used anti-influenza drug.

What fruit extract is it? It's the alkalizing…

Elderberry extract and it is an effective and natural way to reinforce what your immune system is programmed to do: attack the intruders. Florida researchers tested an extract of elderberry fruit in a test tube and observed that the extract of elderberry flavonoids bound directly to the parts of the H1N1 virus that connect with a host. This means that the elderberry extract blocked the viruses' ability to infect more host cells.

In their own words, the researchers concluded that,

"The H1N1 inhibition activities of the elderberry flavonoids compare favorably to the known anti-influenza activities of Tamiflu;"[1]

But the effects of elderberry have a much wider scope that just the H1N1 virus, since it also inhibits certain bacteria and influenza A and B viruses. Last year, German scientists were able to explain this. They observed that the anthocyanins in elderberry enhance immune function because they boost the production of cytokines, which help regulate the immune response.

Tamiflu's Terrible Side Effects

Take a look at the drug's side effects:

- nausea, vomiting, diarrhea
- dizziness, headache, vertigo
- nosebleed
- eye redness or discomfort
- sleep problems (insomnia)
- rash, dermatitis, urticaria, serious skin reactions
- cough or other respiratory symptoms

Notice the irony of the similarity between many of the flu's symptoms and the drug's side effects. But it gets worse, because Tamiflu has other side effects, that although rare, include confusion, delirium, hallucinations, anxiety, unusual behavior, and self-injury. https://www.rxlist.com/tamiflu-side-effects-drug-center.htm

In stark contrast…

Elderberry Extract is a Safe Alternative

At the first symptoms of the flu or even a cold, you can take Elderberry extract without having to worry about side effects. However, be aware that it has a slight diuretic effect, so check with your health practitioner if you take diuretics. Also, the extract lowers blood glucose, so take this into account if you're a diabetic.

You should only use the extract of Sambucus nigra, and never the Sambucus ebulus, since the latter can toxic. And make sure you get the extract from a reputable source, since raw or unripe elderberry, and also the leaves, seeds, and bark, contain cyanide.

The elderberry extract I now have in my winter "First Aid Kit" is alcohol-free, and therefore, it's not acidifying. Many health food stores carry it. If you need to use it, just follow the instructions on the bottle. You should be able to find alcohol-free elderberry extract at most health food stores, or you can order it from an online retailer.

So now you know what to do if you get the flu this year.

https://www.npscript.com/dougcaporrino/sambucus-black-elderberry-syrup/IT0072PAR#undefined2

https://www.npscript.com/dougcaporrino/kids-black-elderberry-syrup/GA0890PAR

Nitric Oxide – Superhero of the Human Body

The chemical inner workings of the human body are sometimes truly amazing. One of the most important examples of this is nitric oxide. This simple molecule has gotten a lot of popular press over the last two decades and for good reason. Nitric oxide provides more health benefits to the human body than just about anything else.

The nitric oxide molecule is a gas and each molecule of this gas is made from one molecule of nitrogen combining with one molecule of oxygen. Scientists and the medical community usually abbreviate nitric oxide as simply NO. The human body produces nitric oxide by utilizing the nitrogen in L-arginine and L-citrulline, both amino acids found in our food.

Nitric oxide serves many functions in the human body. It can act as a messenger between cells, a neurotransmitter, and a hormone.

Nitric oxide benefits:

- helps dilate blood vessels
- supports a healthy heart
- boosts brain power
- improves sexual health

- increases blood flow
- regulates digestion
- increases cognitive abilities
- increases memory retention
- lowers blood pressure
- strengthens the immune system
- increases stamina
- helps re-build muscles after exercise
- increases sex drive
- helps the liver and pancreas function efficiently

Nitric oxide is one busy molecule!

It turns out that nitric oxide is so important to the healthy functioning human systems, it was named "The 1992 Molecule of the Year" by one of the most prestigious scientific journals, "Science." In fact, the Nobel Prize for medicine and physiology was awarded to two scientists in 1998 for their important discovery that the nitric oxide molecule is important for creating signals between nerves and blood vessel cells in the cardiovascular system. Their pioneer work clearly showed that nitric oxide is needed by the body to prevent heart attacks and strokes. More specifically, they found that nitric oxide signals to the lining of blood vessels and capillaries to relax.

Foods that are high in nitric oxide

The foods highest in the raw materials, namely nitrate, needed by the human body to synthesize nitric oxide are **green leafy vegetables** and certain tubers. **Spinach** has one of the very highest concentrations of nitrate as do **beets and beet greens**. It is interesting to note that spinach and beets are in the same plant family! So, as it turns out, Popeye's favorite food really can make you strong!

When it comes to nitric oxide, there are other important dietary considerations. Eating more antioxidants, especially vitamin C and vitamin E, can help prevent the breakdown of nitric oxide in the body. If you are eating greens and beets, you are already getting these antioxidants. However, if you are trying to supplement your diet with a nitric oxide pill, you may not be getting the antioxidants that you need. If you do take a nitric oxide supplement, be sure the supplement contains these important antioxidants. Keep in mind too that the nitrogen content of vegetables varies according to how healthy the soil is. In general, buying organic vegetables will yield more nitrogen available for your body. Another quick point is that **pomegranates** have been found to aid nitric oxide and also to prevent the destruction of nitric oxide so these would be good to add to your diet.

Cardiovascular exercise is an important component of stimulating the body to produce adequate amounts of nitric oxide. Twenty minutes of cardiovascular exercise three to four times a week should be enough to keep the body producing enough nitric oxide. Remember, cardiovascular exercise can be as simple as a brisk walk or even making love!

Another fascinating fact that has been discovered about nitric oxide production in the human body has to do with the commensal anaerobic bacteria found in the biofilm of your tongue and in your saliva. It turns out that when you eat foods high in nitrates like beets and spinach, nitrate becomes concentrated in your mouth. In fact, the mouth contains ten times more nitrate than any other part of your body. The commensal bacteria in your mouth help convert nitrate to nitrite which is then converted to nitric oxide. This explains why taking L-arginine and L-citrulline pills don't work very well. If you quickly swallow a pill, the contents of the pill don't have a chance to interact with these commensal bacteria. Taking slow-dissolving tablets or lozenge is your best bet. Your saliva and the beneficial bacteria in your mouth convert the nutrients in the lozenge into nitric oxide. So, with every swallow, you get a boost of nitric oxide. So, if you would like to supplement nitric oxide, try this product which I have found to be very bioavailable for the body.

https://www.npscript.com/dougcaporrino/nitric-oxide-ultra-capsules/PU0968PAR

Benefits of MSM

About MSM

Technically, MSM is an abbreviation for methyl-sulfonyl-methane, which is organic sulfur compound. This compound is the third largest nutrient found in the human body. MSM is also an ingredient found in quite a few foods, meat, dairy products as well as vegetables.

5 key benefits

From increasing your energy levels to helping with conditions like allergies and asthma, MSM performs a series of important functions in your body every day. Let's look closely at some of the most important ones.

1. Key source of sulfur

Sulfur is perhaps one of the most important nutrients required by our body as it is present in the amino acids which are in turn the basic building blocks of protein. It also has a series of other healing and preventive properties for the human body. MSM happens to be the best form of sulfur which can be consumed both in the form of food products as well as dietary supplements.

2. Bone and joint care

MSM is a beneficial nutrient for your bone health, helping conditions like arthritis, rheumatoid arthritis and osteoarthritis. Being a calcium phosphate dissolver, MSM helps in breaking up the unhealthy calcium deposits in the body that are the root cause of degenerative diseases.

In addition, taking adequate supplements of MSM helps in:

- Improving joint flexibility
- Reducing pain and swelling
- Reducing stiffness
- Improving circulation
- Improving cell vitality

3. The detoxification effect

MSM considerably increases the permeability of your cells which means that it increases cells capability of flushing out excess fluids and toxins. This mechanism has a very important detoxifying effect, making way for essential nutrients into your system and thereby improving the overall functioning of your cell membranes.

4. Skin and hair care

The sulfur provided by MSM produces generous quantities of collagen and keratin, both of which are vital for healthy hair and nails. In fact, MSM is often referred to as the 'beauty mineral' owing to its ability to add to enhance the thickness and strength of nails as well as hair in a very short span of time.

Moreover, research also shows that MSM is quite helpful in the treatment of skin conditions such as:

- Psoriasis
- Eczema
- Rosacea
- Dermatitis
- Acne
- Dandruff

5. Natural energy booster

I just explained how MSM increases the permeability of our cells. Owing to this increased permeability, these cells then need a lesser amount of energy to deal with the accumulated toxins. Moreover, due to the detoxification, it becomes easier for the body to absorb nutrients, which in turn reduces the amount of energy spent on digestion of your food.

Other benefits

- Helps in conditions like asthma
- Helpful in allergies
- Helpful in maintaining a proper pH balance
- Helps cure gastrointestinal issues such as diarrhea, nausea, constipation and hyperacidity
- Helps reduce snoring, when taken diluted with 16 percent water content
- Helps conditions like cramps, headaches and muscular pain, especially caused by hormonal imbalances
- Heals carpal tunnel syndrome
- Helps balance your blood sugar level
- Reduces overall stress levels

Adding on to the vast array of benefits, there is now latest research to show that MSM can also help in warding off the onset of breast cancer. Experiments showed its considerable impact on delaying the development of cancer in animals, almost equivalent to 10 years in human beings.

Similar studies also demonstrate the powerful impact of MSM in suppressing triple-negative breast cancer. In fact, evidence points to the possibility of a potent dose of MSM being capable of reducing the impact of breast cancer in as less as 30 days.

https://www.npscript.com/dougcaporrino/msm-1000mg/DF0084PAR?skuID=DF0084

The Power of the Nap

Sleep is essential part of our overall health. It has always been said that a good eight hours' worth of sleep is the optimum amount for good health and feeling rested – but new studies undertaken in Georgetown University show that this is not necessarily the case. Many scientists are now suggesting that a shorter sleep at night, coupled with a nap during the day, might be the best way to get enough rest and still allow your brain to work at its best.

New studies have shown that even very short naps can significantly enhance cognitive function. The Texas Brain and Spine Institute believes that someday we may be able to harness the positive effect that sleep has on brain function, and by studying these effects we can get closer to improving our health and lifestyle.

The results of this current study have been presented at the 2012 Neuroscience Conference in New Orleans, and they show that by monitoring the brain processes of napping adults, they could determine which parts of the brain are most active. By considering what we know about the brain's division of labor, researchers at the university have determined that taking a nap may have considerably beneficial results in aiding memory loss, blood pressure and other health problems.

In right handed people (or 95% of the population and 13 of the 15 monitored nappers) the left hemisphere of the brain-the one involved in analysis, mathematics and language processing – is generally far more active, while for left handed people it is the right hemisphere – the side concerned with visualization and creative activities – that comes to the fore.

The fact of the right side being considerably more active than the left during napping suggests that naps are actually incredibly good for the brain, allowing it to do the "housework" of clearing space for new memories and new information, so it can effectively process it.

The Mayo Clinic sums it up by stating that we are exposed to a lot of information and that if we are able to sleep on it, the sleep seems to facilitate the transfer of information from the short-term memory bank into the more permanent memory bank.

There are a great many **advantages to taking a nap** than simply waking up feeling slightly more refreshed:

- Studies show that taking a nap can actually **improves memory function**, as the brain can only process so much information before needing to recharge with sleep.
- Taking a nap **clears the brain** of events earlier in the day, and may even help people to process and deal with them more effectively.
- A nap may help to **lower blood pressure**, helping **reduce the risks of heart problems**.
- Napping **reduces stress**.

If you are one of the thousands of people who drink another cup of coffee instead of resting, it may be time to rethink your strategy. Coffee may help keep you awake, but can actually decrease your memory performance, and make you more prone to making mistakes. Taking a nap is far better for your whole body and your brain.

To get the very most out of your catnap, follow these simple tips from:

- Keep your napping regular and stick to a schedule.
- The best time to nap is between 1pm and 3pm, so keep time aside if you can.

- Set an alarm to wake you after 30 minutes or less, anymore and you may wake up groggy.
- Draw the curtains and reduce light as much as you can, as this will make you fall asleep quicker.

Keep warm-your body loses heat during sleep so wrap up in a blanket before you doze off.

Butter or Margarine?

Margarine was originally manufactured to fatten turkeys. When it killed the turkeys, the people who had put all the money into the research wanted a payback so they put their heads together to figure out what to do with this product to get their money back.

It was a white substance with no food appeal so they added the yellow coloring and sold it to people to use in place of butter. How do you like it? They have come out with some clever new flavorings....

DO YOU KNOW. The difference between margarine and butter?

Listen on to the end...gets very interesting!

Both have the same number of calories.

Butter is slightly higher in saturated fats at 8 grams; compared to 5 grams for margarine.

Eating margarine can increase heart disease in women by 53% over eating the same amount of butter, according to a recent Harvard Medical Study.

Eating butter increases the absorption of many other nutrients in other foods.

Butter has many nutritional benefits where margarine has a few and only because they are added!

Butter tastes much better than margarine and it can enhance the flavors of other foods.

Butter has been around for centuries where margarine has been around for less than 100 years.

And now, for Margarine.

Very High in Trans fatty acids.

Triples risk of coronary heart disease ...

Increases total cholesterol and LDL (this is the bad cholesterol) and lowers HDL cholesterol, (the good cholesterol)

Increases the risk of cancers up to five times.

Lowers quality of breast milk

Decreases immune response.

Decreases insulin response.

And here's the most disturbing fact... HERE IS THE PART THAT IS VERY INTERESTING!

Margarine is but ONE MOLECULE away from being PLASTIC... and shares 27 ingredients with PAINT.

These facts alone were enough to have me avoiding margarine for life and anything else that is hydrogenated (this means hydrogen is added, changing the molecular structure of the substance).

Open a tub of margarine and leave it open in your garage or shaded area. Within a couple of days, you will notice a couple of things:

* no flies, not even those pesky fruit flies will go near it (that should tell you something)

* it does not rot or smell differently because it has no nutritional value; nothing will grow on it. Even those teeny weeny microorganisms will not a find a home to grow.

Why? Because it is nearly plastic. Would you melt your Tupperware and spread that on your toast?

Juicing Vs Blending

Juicing and blending offers a simple and effective way of increasing your intake of vegetables and fruits, but they are not the same.

Juicing

Juicing involves extracting all the nutrients in the form of juice from fruits and vegetables minus the pulp, or fiber.

Pros of Juicing

1. **An easy way of obtaining essential vitamins, nutrients, and antioxidants:** Juice provides you with nutrients in an easy, digestible form. To get all the essential nutrients present in a combination of fruits and/or vegetables, all you have to do is place them in your juicer, run the juicer, and drink the produce. Eating all the ingredients in their solid form, on the other hand, would require considerable amount of time, not to mention drive and effort.
2. **It is easy on your digestive system:** Juice does not contain pulp, which, although essential, slows the digestive system. To digest a glass of juice, your digestive system does not have to work as hard to digest the nutrients. This inherent quality of juice is extremely

beneficial to people with a sensitive digestive system or who have certain illness that prevents their digestive system from processing pulp properly.

3. **Provides instant energy:** As juice is absorbed into the blood stream more quickly than solid fruits and vegetables, it is able to provide energy instantly.
4. **Boosts the immune system:** Juices are rich in antioxidants, minerals, and vitamins. These substances improve your immunity function besides reducing toxicity.

- Cons of Juicing

1. **Juices are not a replacement for a meal:** Juices provides instant energy instead of a steady release of energy. Due to this reason, you are likely to feel hungry quickly after you have gulped a glass of antioxidant-rich juice.
2. **Juices can cause spike in the blood sugar levels:** As mentioned above, juices are assimilated into the blood stream almost instantly. While this provides instant energy, it can also increase your blood sugar levels alarmingly.
3. **Juices do not contain fiber:** Besides preventing spike in blood sugar levels, fiber is necessary for a healthy digestive system. When you drink juice, you do not get this essential substance.
4. **Certain fruits and vegetables do not mix well with each other:** Our digestive system processes different fruits and vegetables differently. So, if you are using a combination of different fruits and/or vegetables, ensure that you are aware of which goes with which.

Blending

Blending is an act of creating a thick liquid solution out of vegetables and fruits with all their ingredients, including fiber, intact. Blended concoctions, like juices, offer several health benefits.

- Pros of Blending

1. **It is a complete meal:** Unlike juice, a blended solution is a complete meal as it contains all the ingredients of the produce. A blend of vegetables and/or fruits contains fiber, which experts believe may be effective in reducing the risk of diabetes and heart disease. Fiber, as mentioned earlier, offers other benefits as well, like filling you better and improving the digestive system.
2. **Doesn't cause a spike in blood sugar levels:** Unlike juices, smoothies provide energy at a steady rate and obviate the risk of a sudden increment in blood sugar levels.
3. **Aids digestion:** Consuming foods in liquid form is easier on the digestive system. Moreover, it saves time. If your excuse for not eating enough green vegetables or fruits was lack of time, now you know exactly what you must do—bring home a blender, or conjure up another excuse!
4. **Increases your intake of vegetables and fruits:** Often, we do not eat fruits and vegetables that we do not find tasty. The result of this deliberate abstinence is that we do not get the benefits that foods in our I-don't-like-its-taste list provide. Blending, like juicing, is an effective solution to this problem. You can mix fruits and vegetables that rub your taste buds in the wrong way with items that you like to produce a concoction that is both tasty and healthy.
5. **Ease of clean up:** Compared to juicers, blenders are easier to clean—an additional reason for you to imbibe smoothies.

Cons of Blending

1. **Not ideal when you require instant energy:** Blended concoction releases energy slowly much like solid foods and, as such, is not ideal when you are in need of instant energy, for instance after a workout.
2. **May not be suitable if you have some digestive problem:** If you have a digestive problem that makes it difficult for you to digest fiber, you are better off drinking juices.

To Conclude:

Blending and juicing are not interchangeable, nor are they comparable because they are inherently different from each other. The question which is better, although repeatedly asked, is ill directed as both offer unique benefits. It is not about choosing one over another, but adding them both to your diet. Why choose one over another when you can have them both, and that too to your heart's content.

Raspberry Ketones and Weight Loss Review of Research

What are raspberry ketones and do they work? Well, if you watch the Dr. Oz Show, you may have heard Dr. Oz call raspberry ketones *"The #1 miracle in a bottle to burn your fat."* Since he made that bold statement, I've heard that raspberry ketone supplements are sold so fast that vitamin stores can't keep them on the shelves! So, what I'd like to do is by review the raspberry ketone research — minus the hype that you have already heard about. Only in this way can you make an informed decision about whether raspberry ketones are right for you.

What are raspberry ketones?

Red raspberry ketones are one of many compounds in raspberries and are what gives raspberries their unique smell. Like all things that come from fruits and vegetables, raspberries contain a lot of substances that are healthy —including anthocyanins, vitamin C and beta carotene. As such, **raspberry ketones are also antioxidant.**

Raspberry ketones also "look" similar to **synephrine** and capsicum — two ingredients that have been used in many weight loss supplements over the years such as the **fat burner promoted by Jillian Michaels.** This similarity is likely why scientists considered raspberry ketones as a weight loss agent itself.

Weight loss supplements that contain raspberry ketones include **QuickTrim** — the Kim Kardashian supplement —and **Apidexin.**

Ketone trivia. The name *ketone* is a chemistry term. That's not important. I just thought people might like to know where the word came from. On some websites they spell ketone as "keytone" but this is an incorrect spelling of the word. Again, not important.

Tip. Keep in mind as you read this review that raspberry ketones are not the same thing as ketones that are made when people go on **low-carb** diets or in people who are **diabetic**. Those ketones are not the same as raspberry ketones.

Raspberry ketones and weight loss

When Dr. Oz asked his fitness expert, Lisa Lynn (more about her below) on TV, how she found out about the weight loss properties of raspberry ketones, Lisa said *"Research research research."* So**,** I looked up the research on raspberry ketones and this is what I discovered.

Study #1. In a study published in 2005, called **the Anti-Obesity Action of Raspberry Ketone**, raspberry ketones were given to mice that were fed a high-fat diet for several weeks. Mice were split into different groups, each getting the same calories but getting different amounts of raspberry ketones (either 0.5%, 1% or 2%).

The diets were about 40% fat in each group. Researchers noted that raspberry ketones — that made up between **1% and 2% of total calories** — caused a reduction in body weight and fat buildup in the livers of mice after 10 weeks of use, compared to mice that only were fed a high-fat diet.

Norepinephrine (also called nor-adrenaline) is a brain chemical that can do many things, one of which includes helping to burn fat. This study also incubated isolated mouse fat cells in norepinephrine along with raspberry ketones to see what would happen.

The researchers observed that the combination of raspberry ketones and norepinephrine caused more fat to leave the fat cells than norepinephrine alone.

This is why Dr. Oz said raspberry ketones cause fat cells to shrink.

I'm telling you this because various websites claim that raspberry ketones increase levels of norepinephrine. However, this study did not show that.

Rather, the researches only showed that raspberry ketones **appeared to improve** the fat-burning ability of norepinephrine.

This is actually a good thing because too much norepinephrine can be bad. For example: norepinephrine can raise blood pressure.

Oddly, this study noted that while a 1% intake of raspberry ketones tended to **raise triglyceride** levels in the mice, eating it at a concentration of 5% of total calories tended to reduce triglycerides.

These researchers also quoted previous studies noting that raspberry ketones raised metabolic rates—in rats. That's interesting, but where's the proof that raspberry ketones raise metabolism in people?

So, this was just a mouse study —and a small study at that! Each group only had **6 mice**.

Also, if we really want to be technical, in this study, all the **mice were *male***. What about female mice? Would raspberry ketones have the same weight loss effects in female mice —or more importantly —**women**?

Study #2. In this study, published in 2010, researchers found that red **raspberry ketones inhibited weight gain and improved fat burning** in mice that were fed a high fat diet. Researchers also noted that raspberry ketones increase levels of a hormone made in fat cells.

Dr. Oz said that hormone was *the "hormone that tricks the body into thinking it's thin."* When we put on weight, we reduce the ability of the hormone to work. Sounds good, but red raspberries have only been shown to reduce this hormone **in mice.** What about people? Have raspberry ketone supplements been proven to help people lose weight by raising hormone levels? Nope. Not yet.

So, what's the evidence for raspberry ketones and weight loss? **Only two mouse studies!** Remember, this is the product that Dr. Oz called "*The #1 miracle in a bottle to burn your fat*" Really Dr. Oz? Would you recommend that your patients try a therapy that is only based on 2 mouse studies? I know you wouldn't.

Come on Dr. Oz. Who is doing your research on supplements?

8 Things You Need to Know About Intermittent Fasting

Intermittent fasting, also known as "IF", is an eating pattern that involves alternating between fasting and non-fasting. The most obvious benefit of intermittent fasting is calorie restriction, which studies have shown to improve longevity. However, long life is not the only benefit of this way of eating, it also improves overall health and, by extension, the quality of life.

Most popular intermittent fasting is 16/8 scheme. The numbers 16 and 8 stand for the fast and feast durations, so you fast for 16 hours and feast for 8. Most opt to break the fast at 12:00PM and eat until 8:00PM, but you can move the eight-hour window to better fit your lifestyle. The key is to be consistent, so if you pick 12:00PM – 8:00PM, stick with it daily.

Studies link caloric restriction to increased longevity

Over the years, several scientific studies have proven that reduced caloric intake increases longevity in animals. In one such study, scientists found that rodents lived for almost twice, as long when their food intake was reduced severely. Another elaborate study involving rhesus monkeys, which are closely related to humans, reveals that reduced caloric intake improved resistance to cancer, age-related decline in cognitive abilities, and heart disease besides increasing longevity.

Before we look into some of the most important benefits of intermittent fasting, it is necessary that we get past some of the common myths surrounding it once and for all.

What is not true about intermittent fasting?

- **It entails several days of fasting at one go**

Many fear intermittent fasting involves going without sustenance or food for several days at a stretch. This fear is baseless. Intermittent fasting, at the most, involves a fasting period of 24 hours, during which you can have one main meal. If this appears challenging to you, you can adopt an intermittent fasting protocol that involves shorter fasting period.

- **It is just a fad and its benefits are not scientifically proven**

Above, we saw a couple of scientific studies that support the positive claims made by the proponents of intermittent fasting. We will see results of more scientific studies later when we discuss the benefits of intermittent fasting. So, the claim that benefits of intermittent fasting are not backed by scientific studies is wrong and baseless.

As far as consigning intermittent fasting to 'just-another-new-fad' list goes, the following news, published on several websites, should end the debate permanently: NASA has revealed that it is contemplating exploring fasting as a means for improving the cognitive functioning of its pilots.

- **You should not exercise during the fasting period of an intermittent fasting program**

Counterintuitive as it may appear, moderate exercise for 40 to 50 minutes accentuates the benefits of intermittent fasting.

With common myths explored, let us now take a look at it's the many benefits of intermittent fasting:

Benefits of intermittent fasting

1. Weight loss

As you may know, glucose, or sugar in the blood, is the fuel source of our body. However, during fasting state, when glucose is not available, the body gets fuel by burning fat. This, needless to say, promotes weight loss.

It is necessary to understand that the short periods of fasting do not involve any breakdown of muscle tissue. Contrary to it, the muscle-molding hormone is produced in greater amounts during a fasting state. So, you stand to gain more benefits from a strength training exercise program if you exercise during your fasting state. Similarly, weight loss enthusiasts can increase their body's fat-burning potential by doing moderate cardio exercise during fasting periods.

A Note: If you are new to intermittent fasting, you are more likely to binge on high-caloric food during the eating period following a fasting period. While the tendency to binge after the end of a fasting period is natural, the pattern can be counterproductive. Mindful eating during your eating period can help you curb your binging tendencies, allowing you to get the maximum benefit from your intermittent program. Mindful eating, in short, entails following components: knowing that you have the power to choose the type of food you want to eat, exercising this power all the time, valuing quality over quantity, eating slowly and becoming aware of the sensual capacity of food, and becoming aware of your personal triggers for mindless eating.

Moderate exercise, strength training, cardio, or a combination of both, for reasonable duration – 40 to 60 minutes – during fasting state is safe and beneficial but not intense exercising or exercising for extremely long duration.

2. Prevents Cancer

According to the research conducted by the *Mount Sinai hospital, Chicago, the University of Southern California*, and *the University of California at Berkeley*, the act of fasting may kill cancer cells as well as precancerous cells – cells that lead to cancer.

During the fasting state, the cancer and precancerous cells are not able to get the fuel they require to grow and survive – glucose. Fasting, it is believed, starves cancer and precancerous cells to death.

3. Increases longevity and protects against neurodegenerative diseases

According to the *National Institute on Aging,* fasting promotes neutral activity in the brain that improves our response to degeneration from aging and stroke. A few studies have also hinted that ketones – chemical compounds formed when the body needs to burn fat – produced during fasting may reduce the risk of neurodegenerative diseases such as modern autism, epilepsy, and Alzheimer's.

Warning: Intermittent fasting is recommended to healthy adults. It is always best to consult your doctor before starting on intermittent fasting. Do not adopt an intermittent fasting program if you have health problems, such as diabetes, hypertension, cardiovascular disease, or if you are pregnant.

————————

Propolis: A Natural Antibiotic

For thousands of years, propolis has played a role in the health of humanity. In the days of Hippocrates, propolis was used to heal open sores and ulcers, including internal ones. In ancient Egypt, propolis was used in the process of mummification. In Europe, propolis was said to relieve inflammation and fever, and in World War II it was used to dress wounds sustained in battle.

Over the years, it's been used to fight tuberculosis, colitis, viruses (including the flu virus), and even acne. It's been shown to be effective against harmful bacteria including staphylococcus. It's also been used to enhance the immune system, which makes it doubly effective as an antibiotic – not only does it kill germs; it also boosts your own germ-fighting capabilities.

Components called phytotonizides play a role in propolis' ability to enhance the immune system, as they appear to stimulate phagocytosis.

Propolis can be taken as a supplement to fight bacterial infections. Studies against placebos have shown good results with 500 mg of propolis, so look for this dosage in a supplement, preferably in capsule form.

Because propolis is so effective against inflammation – particularly inflammation of the mucous membranes in the mouth and throat – it is especially useful in cases of sore throat, canker sores, and ulcers.

A study conducted by the Harvard School of Dental Medicine showed propolis to be effective against canker sores. The safe treatment and prevention of painful canker sores has frustrated modern medicine for some time, and this study, done on two groups of patients (one group took propolis supplements and the other group took a placebo) shows propolis not only reduced the number of canker sore outbreaks significantly, but it also improved the patients' quality of life. In other words, they just felt better!

A 2001 study2 showed that propolis has antifungal activity against multiple strains of yeast, including Candida albicans, which causes yeast infections in people. The study showed that propolis was especially effective at fighting fungal infections of the mouth, particularly in denture wearers.

CAUTION: Propolis and Allergies

If you have known allergies to bees, bee products such as honey, or allergies to conifers, poplars, balsams, and/or salicylates, do not use propolis. In addition, some researchers are of the opinion that propolis may aggravate asthma. So, if you have asthma, do not use propolis without first consulting with your doctor. And when in doubt, a consultation with a qualified health professional is in order.

https://www.npscript.com/dougcaporrino/bee-propolis-standardized/PL0056PAR#undefined1

Future of Medicine – Reshaped!

Science is on the move to prove that missing body parts may not be as much of a concern as one thought earlier.

Tissues that were lost, cells that were never there – missing body parts is never good news whether it's a newborn child or someone grown-up. But science seems to be taking huge leaps forward to take care of such concerns. Using tissue regeneration, body parts that never existed are being created. Take the example of a new study by researchers at the Cornell University. Here's what they found.

A new ear is possible

In the study, scientists proved that it is indeed possible to print out body parts. They did this by creating a new ear using a 3-D printer and living cell injections. Researchers used cow cartilage – more easily available than human cartilage apart from being more flexible – to craft the new ear. The next step is now to be able to cultivate a child's ear cartilage in a way that the regenerated ear can fill in the spots that are missing. Researchers linked to the study are working on this. Through this study and forthcoming research, scientists are trying to prove that technology has come to a point where it can be used to create 3-D structures and that the latter can come into the mainstream over a period of time.

To make the ear a reality, researchers first used a 3-D camera to capture images of a child's ear. The camera was made to move around the child's head to produce images that could later be used to confirm a match with the real ear. The images taken, a 3-D printer came into the picture to create an exact soft mold of the original ear. The mold was then injected with a collagen gel containing animal collagen. Next, about 250 million cartilage cells were injected into the ear. The collagen acted as a scaffold on which the ear cells eventually grew.

Later, the researchers put the ear into a cell culture medium for about three to five days before implanting it. In the next three months following this, the cartilage cells were at work constantly. At the end of that period, cartilage was able to replace collagen completely, resulting in what appeared to be a workable outer ear. The scientists are now just waiting for the day when a patient's own cells will become a major contributor in the process.

Now that a new ear can be created, parents of children born without ears or born with malformed ears can breathe a sigh of relief. In fact, this development can be an advantage to anyone looking for customized implants. This study is a feather on the cap of tissue regeneration – something that has been gaining prominence significantly – but it's not the first of its kind.

Healing wounds becomes quicker

The Wake Forest School of Medicine situated in North Carolina in association with the Armed Forces Institute of Regenerative Medicine came up with a technique to "print" skin cells on burn wounds. For this project, researchers used a laser printer to scan the burn wound so that a precise map can be created. This map was later used during the printing process so that the printer had ready directions on where to place the cells. Instead of cartridges, the researchers used vials to contain the cells and print them directly on to the wound.

The experiment came as a result of the present scenario in wound healing. Though there are skin substitutes available in the market, the size is still limited. And even under circumstances where a workable skin substitute is found, the latter usually takes a long time to be prepared.

Burn wounds are also widely treated with skin grafts. However, this traditional method has a major problem: burn victims often don't have enough skin left unharmed skin to harvest these grafts. The 3-D skin printing technique, in such cases, can work wonders. Researchers found out that the technique not only promotes quick healing, but also stabilizes the wound faster.

Heart tissues and blood vessels get repaired

In 2008, the Tissue Engineering journal carried a report about how researchers at the University of Missouri had been able to print cardiac tissue as well as blood vessels. During the study, researchers printed cardiac cells and incubated them for 70 hours. This led to the cells fusing together to form tissue that began beating like any other heart tissue after about 90 hours. Similarly, heart valves, knee cartilage, and bone implants have also been successfully printed by a team of bio-engineers at Cornell University. In these experiments, the experts have extracted cells from the corresponding part of the patient's body. That apart, they've also created a special ink to print these body parts.

3-D printing has already made a mark in the world of medicine. The wait is now to see how it reshapes our future.

Phytoplankton – Super Food of The Future

The oceans of the earth contain the largest concentration of life on this planet and life on earth revolves around the oceans. The greatest numbers of organisms on the oceans are tiny forms of animal and plant life collectively known as the "plankton', which is a Greek word for "wanderer" or "drifter, as they drift in the water._All plankton are inert floaters and do not actively swim in the water, however, they are the most numerous organisms in the oceans - and clearly the most important as well. In fact, the marine phytoplankton (phyto=plant) release vital oxygen into the atmosphere and inhabit the pivotal base of the ecosystem. These minute organisms can be considered to be the basis of all ecosystems and one of the most vital organisms when the Earth is taken as one planetary biological arena. The billions of phytoplankton in the oceans form the very basis of life on this world, a vital link in the chain of life as many processes in the environment are affected by their life cycles. The billions of tiny organisms in the oceans play an important role in the carbon cycle of the oceans and are food sources forming the very bottom of the food chain of planet earth. Huge volumes of carbon dioxide from the atmosphere are absorbed and utilized by the phytoplankton in the oceans with the resultant release of oxygen into the atmosphere - oxygen is the very basis of all animal life. Thus, the phytoplankton in the oceans is necessary for all life in the world.

Phytoplankton in the oceans can be seen as microscopic powerhouse plants that produce concentrated raw materials and release them into the food chain; they also release and store essential minerals as well as varied nutritional compounds that are necessary to the maintenance of cellular health in a biological system.

CELLS AND LIFE

The cellular arena is the foundation of all life on the planet, and every function of the biological body is dependent on the biochemical mechanisms operant in the cells. Indeed, all the crucial tasks and the metabolic actions of a body take place in the cells forming the organism.

Cells are autonomous systems that absorb nutrients and convert them into something else; they are also responsible for the disposal of the various toxins produced as a result of chemical reactions. All the metabolic energy required for every mental and physical function of an organism is produced in the cell. The vital functioning of an organism is based on the communication existing in between cells, which are constantly transmitting and receiving signals from one another, thus uniting the entire organism as a whole. The cellular arena is also responsible for numerous other functions that make up a living system - storage, protection, sensory activities, etc. This is why cellular health always translates into general health in the entire body.

Like all other plants on planet earth, all the phytoplankton's manufacture their own food using sunlight and carbon dioxide, and water - releasing oxygen as a byproduct. Therefore, all the phytoplankton of the world are photosynthetic that synthesize their own edible organic substances (photo is light, synthesis is built). These minute life forms contain concentrated amounts of the vital food manufacturing green pigments known as chlorophyll - this pigment is the principal agent required for natural photosynthesis to take place. The production of organic end products is the goal of photosynthesis; during the process energy containing nutrients called carbohydrates are formed by the plant at the cellular level. The thousands of different species of fishes and other oceanic animals such as whales are dependent on the phytoplankton and zooplankton. Indeed, at the basic level, the plankton is the only nourishment for all marine life. The varied species of phytoplankton are what give fishes the healthy fatty acids called the omega-3 fats - such as (EPA) and (DHA). Humans also benefit from the same omega-3 fatty acids, when they consume fishes in the diet. Human health is boosted by the omega-3 fats, and a diet rich in these fats is very beneficial. Clinical research has confirmed that a greater consumption of these beneficial fatty acids translates into a reduced risk for many forms of cardiovascular diseases, auto-immune disorders as well as behavioral disorders.

PLANKTON FOR HUMAN USE

Human beings can benefit from the nutrients stored by these tiny plants according to results from recent studies - this may be one way in which the world huge human population can find more food to feed its growing population. Indeed, as a source of nutrients, these micro-plants are in the same league as the numerous other beneficial "super green" products that have been in stores for decades now. Phytoplankton may not be simply a fad food, however, as it is potentially valuable as an almost limitless resource for a hungry world.

Some common plant products including sea weeds like kelp, chlorella and spirulina have become quite popular to people wishing to maintain their youthful vigor and overall health in the long term. However, the nutritional quality of phytoplankton is not similar to the nutritional profile of these products.

As far as cellular nutrition and health are concerned, the quality and nature of the nutrients obtained from the food is the single most important factor. Cellular health is also affected by the environment surrounding all cells; this includes the real level of various toxins and external factors such as stress. The consumption of nutrient poor and highly processed food products over a long period of time tends to impact cellular health in a deleterious way. The health of cells is compromised by a poor diet.

At the same time and to add to the problems, the nutrient depleted soils and the poor agricultural practices in the modern age has made it so much more difficult for an individual to gain adequate nutritional benefits from foods. The nutrient levels in whole and unprocessed foods are also low nowadays and this has a telling impact on health. The entire human body tends to be affected when cells are malnourished or damaged - the depletion of any vital nutrient in the cell will immediately register on the functioning of the body as a whole.

HUMAN NUTRITION AND PLANKTON

There are some positive things to say about the human body, it is very resilient. It is capable of healing itself and has a capacity to bounce back from a disease. The human body possesses an innate tendency to heal and regain its balance when all the necessary nutritional elements are found in the diet - therefore, diet and food play an important role in diseases and their treatment. The high nutritional value of plankton is being recognized and some very health - conscious individuals are already turning to marine phytoplankton supplements to boost cellular health. The biochemical metabolic functions of the human body are promoted by the unique blend of phytonutrients found in the phytoplankton. The high nutritional value of phytoplankton is of a very high order, in fact, the entire range of essential trace minerals necessary to the human body are in proportion to what is found in human blood. Therefore, phytoplankton may well be the ideal or the super food of tomorrow.

When analyzed, phytoplankton are found to contain nutrients which are a veritable combination of all the major trace minerals found in the oceans and seas. This trove of essential trace minerals is found along with many other essential cellular nutrients, such as the vital amino acids which make up all the proteins, phytoplankton's are also rich in their content of the omega-3 fatty acids, as well as being rich sources of many vital vitamins, different enzymes and small traces of other micronutrients - all of which are good for human health and nutrition.

The nutritional value of marine phytoplankton's and its beneficial effects on humans is continually being unveiled by food scientists continue in the laboratory. The promise of phytoplankton in nutrition is such that, clinical studies to study its effectiveness as a supplement in dealing with obesity and diabetes have been started in some laboratories around the world.

The functioning of the cellular membranes is supported and boosted by all the vital nutrients that are found in marine phytoplankton, these nutrients also aid metabolism at the cellular level. They are also important as agents bringing about detoxification in the cells. These nutrients also boost the production of energy at the cellular level according to the scientific evidence. As any improvement in the health at a cellular level translates into general health in the body, consuming this super food as a supplement may well be great addition in any nutritional program.

Phytoplankton is a very interesting choice as food choices go, especially when this fish food is to be adapted for the consumption of human beings. The view of most nutritionist is that the consumption of phytoplankton could be a nutritional bonanza, it may have great beneficial effects on cardiovascular health, and it may possibly be useful in dealing with problems such as chronic fatigue syndrome, in dealing with weight loss. The nutrients found in phytoplankton may also help in alleviating blood sugar disorders, and in reducing the impact of arthritis and some serious digestive disorders that are commonly associated with a poor diet. Though, unverified in scientific tests the testimonials associated with the use of phytoplankton supplements are amazing, there are even reports of complete recoveries from disorders that are almost believed to be beyond cure, following the long-term use of these phytoplankton supplements.

PLANKTON SUPPLEMENTS

The American Journal of Clinical Nutrition recently published a review about the health protecting qualities and the benefits of consuming raw fresh fruit and vegetables, the paper linked these beneficial effects of the foods to the complex mixture of photochemical found in the food items - these compounds are also responsible for the variety of colors seen on the skin of fruits and vegetables. Chemists working in the laboratory have confirmed the presence of up wards of five thousand phytochemicals in plant foods - how many types exists unidentified and uncaptioned remains a mystery requiring painstaking study. At the same time, clinical researchers have confirmed convincingly in laboratory tests that many plant pigments and phytochemicals present in foods are capable of working synergistically as antioxidants to fight disease by scavenging free radicals, produced as a result of normal metabolic processes at the cellular level. In fact, many disease states and disorders affecting the human body are believed to be either caused by oxidation at the cellular level - this vital chemical reaction also results in the creation of free radicals - or due to excessive oxidation of metabolites leading to cellular damage. Oxidation describes a negative reaction caused by oxygen that causes the "rusting" of cells, tissues, and organs. These free radicals are very reactive molecules that disrupt cellular machinery and induce disease states by damaging cells. Compounds called antioxidants found mainly in plant based foods can slow down these freewheeling oxidative agents by scavenging the free radicals - neutralizing them chemically. The action of these anti-oxidants prevents any cellular damage and as a result prevents a disease state from affecting the particular cell in question. Large amounts of antioxidant pigments and nutrients are found in the phytoplankton's - this alone is sufficient to encourage their supplemental use in treating disease states.

PLANKTON AND NUTRITION

Food items sourced in their natural state, such as the phytoplankton, contain the full range of nutritional compounds compared to processed food products. The range of nutrients include all the essential vitamins, the important major minerals and the trace minerals, organic compounds like proteins, as well as special compounds like the free radical scavenging antioxidants such as the carotenoids and the omega-3 fatty acids so useful in combating some disease states. The main benefit of whole and raw foods is that the nutrients present in whole foods work synergistically to improve overall health and help maintain the body. The combined effect of the multitude of nutrients found in plant foods is pointed out as being the reason for the health benefits associated with them, according to most nutritionist, the synergistic working of these varied nutrients results in a net positive effect on the body as they balance each other out - the result, is good health for the person consuming such foods. The hopeful term a natural "insurance policy" may be applied to diets that contain a lot of such wholesome plant-based foods. Phytoplankton is a whole nutritional package by itself, filled with all the essential nutrients that can ever be required in the human body. Supplements of phytoplankton are therefore called for to support the daily meals as an extra source of much needed nutrients. Phytoplankton can also be seen as the ideal green food, an alkaline food item that is extremely rich in essential minerals which are organically bound inside the structure making up the plankton. Vital minerals such as calcium, magnesium, potassium and manganese are all found in high amounts in the organic form in phytoplankton and are thus readily absorbed into the body. Therefore, the phytoplankton are complete nutritional foods in themselves.

Unlike any other food, Phytoplankton is being hailed as the new 'super food' as it is 100% nutritionally useful and bio-available to the body; when you eat it, nothing whatsoever gets wasted. Most normal foods like fruits, vegetables, nuts, grains, meat and fish actually contain less than 50% nutritional value that is useful to the body.

During the digestive process humans produce a significant quantity of waste by-products from consuming these conventional foods. These waste by-products produce toxicity and stress in the body, particularly if the gut, liver and other organs are not functioning correctly. Over time, this toxic stress overload can lead to illness and disease, hence the record levels of drugs being prescribed nowadays.

https://www.npscript.com/dougcaporrino/msm-1000mg/DF0084PAR?skuID=DF0084

A Drug Recall That Should Frighten Us All About The FDA

US Food and Drug Administration (FDA) Commissioner Margaret Hamburg

Pay attention, as I can't say this seriously enough. The FDA took a drug off the market, and the reasons should send shivers of fear down the backs of consumers, investors, generic drug companies – and the FDA.

The FDA announced that the 300mg generic version of Wellbutrin XL manufactured by Impax Laboratories and marketed by Teva Pharmaceuticals was being recalled because it did not work. And this wasn't just a problem with one batch – this is a problem that has been going on with this particular drug for four or five years, and the FDA did everything it could to ignore it.

The FDA apparently approved this drug – and others like it – without testing it. The FDA just assumed if one dosage strength the drug companies submitted for approval works, then the other higher dosages work fine also. With this generic, American consumer became the FDA's guinea pigs to see if the FDA's assumption was right. It wasn't.

Background

In December 2006, the first generic versions of the popular anti-depressant Wellbutrin XL were approved by the FDA. The drug comes in two dosage strengths, 150 milligrams and 300mg. The 300mg dose is generally used for patients with more severe depression and anxiety and patients who don't respond to the lower dose. The FDA approved generic versions of both dosage strengths from a few generic drug companies: Teva Pharmaceuticals (manufactured by Impax Laboratories and marketed by Teva Pharmaceuticals), Anchen, Actavis, Watson Pharmaceuticals and Mylan Pharmaceuticals. Almost immediately, the FDA started receiving reports from patients that claimed the 300mg dose was being associated with side effects and reduced efficacy.

The People's Pharmacy, a well-known syndicated radio and newspaper columnist husband and wife team, notified the FDA that hundreds of patients had logged their own complaints of side effects with the then-recently approved generic version of Wellbutrin XL. The FDA brushed off the People's Pharmacy and others that raised the issue, stating that they had faith that the drugs were equivalent and that perhaps the patients, who had mental disease, were more prone to perceived problems with a change in the medication than others. This was seen by many as essentially telling patients "it's all in their head." After several more years and public outcry, the FDA was forced to take-action.

What Action Did the FDA Take?

Instead of doing its own study on the drug, the FDA asked the drug maker to conduct a study to determine whether the generic drug was equivalent to the brand. The FDA, in their recent press release, claims that Teva started the trial but later abandoned it because of slow patient enrollment. It was already 2010, several years after knowing there was a problem, the FDA was forced to do its own study.

Did the FDA Drag Its Heels?

The FDA study was completed in August 2012 – more than 5 years after the initial problems were reported. The FDA study showed that the 300mg dose from Teva is ineffective insomuch as it did not deliver enough of the drug.

Oddly, despite the result being available in August 2012, the public was only made aware of this in October 2012.

How Did This Happen?

When the FDA issued its press release on October 3rd, it said that the FDA made a mistake in that it had taken the data for the 150mg version. Since that dosage had worked fine, the FDA just assumed that the 300mg dosage would work. I am not joking – they indicated that this case caused them to change the way they do things. They approved the drugs by extrapolating the data for the 150mg, assuming the 300mg works the same.

Clearly, the FDA has serious doubts on how they approved the 300mg dosages by just assuming if the 150mg works then the 300mg must work also. The FDA's press release makes that clear:

FDA has approved five generic versions of Wellbutrin XL 300 mg. Each of these generics was approved based on bioequivalence studies comparing the 150 mg strength of the products to Wellbutrin XL 150 mg. **Studies were not performed directly on the 300 mg strength of the products.** Rather, the bioequivalence studies were performed using the 150 mg strength, and the results were extrapolated to establish bioequivalence of the 300 mg product.

FDA has determined that this approach is no longer appropriate to establish bioequivalence of 300 mg bupropion hydrochloride extended-release tablets to Wellbutrin XL 300 mg, and the Agency is revising its guidance to industry for how to conduct premarket bioequivalence studies in generic bupropion products.

This cleverly worded press release hides the fact that this method of approving Wellbutrin XL or any drug is not only "no longer" appropriate, but was never an appropriate way of approving drugs. Just extrapolating data is an erroneous assumption and ignores basic principles known by most high school science students. In addition, if you don't test the larger dosages, what if drug companies simply submitted 300mg drugs that had no drug in them? That seems like more than just a moronic mistake, but a dangerous approach to approving drugs.

How This is A Safety Issue?

The lack of efficacy for a high dose anti-depressant is really a safety issue, not a manufacturing issue.

How many patients who were not adequately treated on the 150mg dose were put on the 300mg only to see their symptoms get worse because the generic did not work as promised? How many patients, doctors, and their families thought that this was simply a further deterioration of a patient's condition and mental state? How many parents had to worry about their children when their anti-depressant seemed to stop working? How many people committed suicide taking a generic antidepressant that did not work?

And the appalling part of all this is that the fact that this could have been prevented if the FDA had simply tested the drug before they approved it, or at the least heeded the hundreds of complaints.

IP6 Treatment for Cancer

Anyone looking for effective alternatives to the treatments offered by traditional cancer specialists might want to look at inositol hexophosphate (IP6). It is a very simple and inexpensive treatment that may easily get written off by people, who have been led to believe the cure for cancer can only be found in a laboratory through the complexities of science and only after years of expensive research and testing. Yet it is becoming obvious that one of the most effective cures for cancer already exists in a simple compound found in abundance in many foods. New research continues to underscore the effectiveness of IP6 against cancer.

IP6 is non-toxic and produces no side effect

IP6 is a compound found in beans, whole grains, nuts, seeds, rice and wheat bran, corn, and sesame. One-half cup of whole kernel corn contains a whopping 650 mgs of IP6. It is composed of an inositol sugar molecule (one of the B vitamins), with six phosphate groups attached. Because it is a sugar molecule, it has a pleasant, sweet taste. Because it is from food and not from a drug laboratory, IP6 has no toxic effects in the body even at high doses.

Although the IP6 compound was identified many years ago, it wasn't until the late 1980's that its ability to control the rate of abnormal cell division was discovered. A scientist from the University of Maryland, found that IP6 was able to halt well developed cancers. While most cancer research centered on killing cancer cells, this DR proved that IP6 could normalize the sugar production of cancerous cells, thereby altering their gene expression toward a more healthful state. This discovery has major implications because cancer cells that are well behaved have far fewer negative consequences to health.

IP6 works in many ways against cancer

Whether from food or from therapeutic supplemental doses, IP6 works against cancer in several ways. Its ability to act as an intracellular messenger means that it is integral in many cellular activities including:

Normalizing the rate of cell growth

When cancer cells lose their control mechanisms, rapid and uncontrolled division of malignant cells is often the result. As IP6 repairs the gene mutations and reestablishes control within the cells, their rate of division is slowed

Enhancing natural killer cells

Natural killer cells are white blood cells that help protect against infected or cancerous cells. Research has shown that the higher the amount of natural killer cell activity, the lower the incidence of some cancers. A healthy human produces 500 to 1000 cancer cells daily that need to be identified and disposed of by the body. Natural killer cells and natural cell programming result in the vast majority of these cells being destroyed and removed. However, when the body is under stress, including the stress produced by lack of sleep, natural killer cell population is compromised. When the body is under the ultimate stress of being forced to face a diagnosis of cancer and the terrifying toxic treatments that go with such a diagnosis, the natural killer cell population can be reduced at the time it is most needed. IP6 has been documented and proven to increase natural killer cells at such times.

Normalizing cell physiology

Because IP6 is able to restore aspects of normality to the cells, it is able to modulate how a cancer cell expresses itself and how threatening it will be. Experiments have shown that IP6 is able to normalize several aspects of cell physiology in spite of the fact that cancer cells have altered DNA. It was demonstrated in the above noted study that IP6 is able to alter gene expression to restore normality. The more a cell can return to its normal state, the more it loses its malignant characteristics.

Powerfully chelating heavy metal

Tumor cells use iron as a primary growth factor. According to researchers at Wake Forest University, iron chelators are of value in the treatment of cancer since they act by depleting iron and limiting tumor growth. IP6 binds with iron and escorts it from the body. Because IP6 is naturally found in all human cells, it has the ability to get inside tumor cells and remove their iron.

Inhibiting metastasis

IP6 inhibits cancer cell migration and invasion by preventing the adhesion of these cells to extra-cellular matrix proteins. This limited adhesion is very important following surgery and biopsy, as these procedures can cause cancer cells to become dislodged. One reason so many breast cancer patients have lymph nodes containing cancer cells is that the squeezing of the breast by the mammography used in diagnosis can dislodge cancer cells which then migrate to the lymph nodes.

In addition to the anti-cancer benefits of IP6, research is revealing its benefits in treating diabetes, depression, osteoporosis, heart disease, and kidney stones. It has recently been shown to help Parkinson's patients because of its ability to chelate excess iron and thereby reduce oxidative stress that results in neuronal degradation.

Treating cancer with IP6

For anyone choosing to use IP6 as a cancer cure or a preventative there are some things to know. IP6 is present in all human cells, and considered quite safe to use. However, IP6 obtained from food is bound to protein. Before it can be absorbed by the body, it must be freed from this protein by the enzyme phytase that is present in food and naturally in the intestinal tract. The power of the phytase enzyme is damaging to IP6 and renders much of it inactive and therefore less effective when obtained in this form. Pure IP6 from a supplement is not bound to protein and is easily absorbed intact and able to provide its complete medicinal properties.

Many holistic healers and naturopaths recommend IP6 as a standard alternative treatment to be used along with others alternative treatments for active cancer. For people with a high risk of cancer or who have had cancer and want to prevent a recurrence, IP6 is also consistently recommended. Some traditional physicians are becoming aware of the benefits of IP6 and although they can't bring themselves to abandon their toxic treatments, they are adding IP6 to their protocols.

https://www.npscript.com/dougcaporrino/ip6-inositol-hexaphosphate-/PU0320PAR

Safety of HPV Vaccine

There are currently two HPV vaccines on the market, but if there was any regard for sound scientific evidence, neither would be promoted as heavily as they are.

The first, Gardasil, was licensed by the US Food and Drug Administration (FDA) in 2006. It is now recommended as a routine vaccination for girls and women between the ages of 9-26 in the US. On October 25, 2011, the CDC's Advisory Committee on Immunization Practices also voted to recommend giving the HPV vaccine to males between the ages of 11 and 21. The second HPV vaccine, Cervarix, was licensed in 2009.

Were it to be discovered that the HPV vaccine, in fact, does not effectively prevent cancer, then young women (and now boys) are being exposed to clearly unacceptable health risks. And that's precisely what a recent study has concluded...

Review of HPV Trials Conclude Effectiveness is Still Completely Unproven

Published online on September 24, a systematic review of pre- and post-licensure trials of the HPV vaccine by a Canadian team shows that its effectiveness is not only overstated (through the use of selective reporting or "cherry picking" data) but also completely *unproven.*

The summary states it quite clearly:

"We carried out a systematic review of HPV vaccine pre- and post-licensure trials to assess the evidence of their effectiveness and safety. We find that HPV vaccine clinical trials design, and data interpretation of both efficacy and safety outcomes, were largely inadequate. Additionally, we note ***evidence of selective reporting of results from clinical trials*** *(i.e., exclusion of vaccine efficacy figures related to study subgroups in which efficacy might be lower or even negative from peer-reviewed publications).*

Given this, the widespread optimism regarding HPV vaccines long-term benefits appears to rest on a number of unproven assumptions (or such which are at odd with factual evidence) and significant misinterpretation of available data.

For example, ***the claim that HPV vaccination will result in approximately 70% reduction of cervical cancers is made despite the fact that the clinical trials data have not demonstrated to date that the vaccines have actually prevented a single case of cervical cancer (let alone cervical cancer death), nor that the current overly optimistic surrogate marker-based extrapolations are justified.***

Likewise, ***the notion that HPV vaccines have an impressive safety profile is only supported by highly flawed design of safety trials and is contrary to accumulating evidence from vaccine safety surveillance databases and case reports which continue to link HPV vaccination to serious adverse outcomes (including death and permanent disabilities).***

We thus conclude that further reduction of cervical cancers might be best achieved by optimizing cervical screening (which carries no such risks) and targeting other factors of the disease rather than by the reliance on vaccines with questionable efficacy and safety profiles."

It's important to realize that the HPV vaccine only protects against a small select set of HPV viruses that can lead to cell abnormalities that in **some** instances can cause cervical cancer, *if the abnormalities are not identified and treated.* So, in reality, it's a misnomer to call it an anti-cancer vaccine. And it's massively misleading, if not a deliberate deception, to claim it "will" save lives.

Today, six years after licensure, we STILL have absolutely *no proof,* not a shred of actual evidence, indicating that Gardasil actually prevents cancer in the long-term and/or reduces cervical cancer mortality.

As of August 13, 2014, VAERS has received 119 reports of death following HPV vaccination, as well as:

- 894 reports of disability
- 517 life-threatening adverse events
- 9,889 emergency room visits
- 2,781 hospitalizations

A Ketogenic Diet for Cancer

A ketogenic diet is one in which carbohydrates, and to a lesser extent, proteins are restricted in the diet and replaced with fat. This treatment has been effective for seizure control in epileptic children for over a century and more recently for the treatment of obesity-related disorders. It may also provide a benefit in cancer subtypes with outcomes closely related to obesity and metabolic risk factors, such as breast cancer. It generally implements a ratio of 4:1 fat to protein and carbohydrates. However, many people will reach significant ketosis when their carbohydrates are limited to less than 50g per day, and others at around 20-30g.

What are Ketones?

Ketones are energy sources produced by our liver that can freely cross our blood brain barrier to provide a source of energy for our neurons (brain cells). These ketones replace glucose when it is not available, such as during fasting, during the winter months in traditional societies.

How Can a Ketogenic Diet Help Cancer Treatment?

Much like most things in cancer, including chemotherapy, biologic agents, and even radiation therapy, we do not quite know exactly how a ketogenic diet works. However, there are several potential mechanisms:

- First and foremost a ketogenic diet may work simply through decreasing available glucose to tumor cells. Many decades ago, Otto Warburg stated that a hallmark of cancer was the uptake of glucose by cancer cells. Cancer cells rely on glucose for energy; therefore, any method of limiting this may help to "starve" cancer cells. Recent data from several universities, including Johns Hopkins have shown that in brain tumors, the higher a patient's blood glucose level, the lower their survival.
- Other data has shown that this occurs due to deficient and defective mitochondria. Since mitochondria can create energy from proteins and fats, this deficiency leaves cancer cells reliant on the breakdown of sugar, for energy. Interestingly, our cells use this process as well, especially when oxygen is not available. This is what occurs in muscle cells during sprinting or lifting heavy weights. Lactic acid is released, resulting in a burning sensation within the muscles. Cancer cells, on the other hand, appear to use glycolysis for energy regardless of whether oxygen is present or not. This process is very inefficient for energy production, and mitochondria can create around 20 times more ATP than the process of glycolysis. A ketogenic diet allows the body to rely on the mitochondria for energy.
- Due to their faulty mitochondria, cancer cells also rely on glucose to fix free radical damage. Much like our normal cells, cancer cells are constantly experiencing bombardment with free radicals, and maybe even more so than our cells. Since their mitochondria do not function properly, they rely on even more uptake of glucose, which is used to counter free radical damage. Limiting this glucose will inhibit their cell damage repair.
- Cancer cells require more than just fuel to survive, much like our normal cells, they use signaling hormones that tell them to

grow and survive. Cancer cells have receptors on them, like the insulin growth factor receptor (IGF-1R). Insulin growth factor (IGF) can bind to this, as can insulin, which is secreted in our bloodstream in response to carbohydrate consumption. Insulin then activates several pathways that increase cancer growth and survival. A recent study in advanced cancer patients confirmed the ability of a ketogenic diet to significantly decrease the insulin pathway in tumor cells.

- Please remember that all cancers are not create equal. Read Dr. Gonzalez's book "**Nutrition and The Autonomic Nervous System - The Scientific Foundations of The Gonzalez Protocol.**" In this book he describes the different types of cancers and the different diets they respond too.

Superbugs Invade American Supermarkets

Antibiotic-resistant bacteria are now common in the meat aisles of American supermarkets. These so-called superbugs can trigger foodborne illness and infections that are hard to treat.

An analysis by the Environmental Working Group has determined that government tests of raw supermarket meat published last February detected antibiotic-resistant bacteria in:

These little-noticed tests, the most recent in a series conducted by the National Antimicrobial Monitoring System, a joint project of the federal Food and Drug Administration, Centers for Disease Control and Prevention and U.S. Department of Agriculture, found that supermarket meat samples collected in 2014 harbored significant amounts of the superbug versions of *salmonella* and *Campylobacter*, which together cause 3.6 million cases of food poisoning a year.

Moreover, the researchers found that some 53 percent of raw chicken samples collected in 2014 were tainted with an antibiotic-resistant form of *Escherichia coli*, or *E. coli*, a microbe that normally inhabits feces. Certain strains of *E. coli* can cause diarrhea, urinary tract infections and pneumonia. The extent of antibiotic-resistant *E. coli* on chicken is alarming because bacteria readily share antibiotic-resistance genes.

Not surprisingly, superbugs spawned by antibiotic misuse — and now pervasive in the meat Americans buy — have become a direct source of foodborne illness. Even more ominously, antibiotic misuse threatens to make important antibiotics ineffective in treating human disease. In the past, people who became ill because of contact with harmful microbes on raw meat usually recovered quickly when treated with antibiotics. But today, the chances are increasing that a person can suffer serious illness, complications or death because of a bacterial infection that doctors must struggle to control.

The proliferation of antibiotic-resistant bacteria poses special dangers to young children, pregnant women, the elderly and people with weakened immune systems.

Among the most worrisome recent developments:

- The federal tests published in February determined that **9 percent** of raw chicken samples and **10 percent** of raw ground turkey sampled from retail supermarkets in 2014 were tainted with a superbug version of salmonella bacteria. Antibiotic resistance in salmonella is growing fast: of all salmonella microbes found on raw chicken sampled in 2014, **74 percent** were antibiotic-resistant, compared to less than 50 percent in 2002. These microbes, frequently found on chicken and turkey and occasionally on beef and pork, commonly cause diarrhea and in extreme cases can lead to arthritis.
- In the same federal tests, a superbug version of the *Campylobacter* microbe was detected on **26 percent** of raw chicken pieces. Raw turkey samples contained numerically fewer of these microbes, but **100 percent** of those examined were antibiotic-resistant. The *Campylobacteria* pathogen is a common cause of diarrhea and in severe cases can trigger an autoimmune disease that results in paralysis and requires intensive care treatment.
- In 2006 FDA scientists found superbug versions of a particularly troublesome strain of *E. coli*, responsible for more than 6 million infections a year in the U.S., on **16 percent** of ground turkey and **13 percent** of chicken. Fully **84 percent** of the *E. coli* bacteria identified in these tests were resistant to antibiotics.

- In its own tests of raw pork, published last January, Consumer Reports magazine found that **63 percent** contained a superbug version of *Yersinia,* a microbe that can cause long-lasting bouts of diarrhea.
- In 2014 tests, researchers at Northern Arizona University and the Translational Genomics Research Institute found that **74 percent** of store-bought raw turkey samples were tainted with bacteria resistant bugs to at least one antibiotic. Of these staph bacteria, **79 percent** were resistant to **three or more** types of antibiotics. Staph can cause skin infections in exposed cuts or that cause foodborne illness.

A significant contributor to the looming superbug crisis, according to scientists and health experts, is **unnecessary** antibiotic usage by factory farms that produce most of the 8.9 million animals raised for food in the U.S. every year. Industrial livestock producers routinely dose their animals with pharmaceuticals, mostly administered with limited veterinary oversight and frequently without prescriptions, to encourage faster growth or prevent infection in crowded, stressful and often unsanitary living conditions.

Overuse of antibiotics in people, often for colds and other viral illnesses, has contributed to antibiotic resistance, too, but responsible doctors generally take care not to prescribe them unnecessarily.

Pharmaceutical makers have powerful financial incentives to encourage abuse of antibiotics in livestock operations. In 2014, they sold nearly 30 million pounds of antibiotics for use on domestic food-producing animals, up 22 % over 2005 sales by weight, according to reports complied by the FDA and the Animal Health Institute, an industry group. Today, pharmaceuticals sold for use on food-producing animals amount to nearly 80% of the American antibiotics market, according to the Pew Campaign on Human Health and Industrial Farming. Pew calculates that the market for antibiotics for treatment of people has been flat for some years, hovering at around 7.7 million pounds annually.

As the superbug problem has exploded into a full-fledged global health crisis, medical authorities worldwide are sounding increasingly urgent alarms.

The federal government's Interagency Task Force warned last year that "drug choices for the treatment of … infections are becoming increasingly limited and expensive, and, in some cases, nonexistent."

Also last year, Dr. Margaret Chan, director general of the World Health Organization, said that if important antibiotics become useless, "things as common as strep throat or a child's scratched knee could once again kill."

Slowing the spread of antibiotic resistance will require concerted efforts, not only by doctors, patients and veterinarians but also livestock producers and big agribusinesses.

Antibiotics, the lifesaving drugs that treat bacterial infections, came into widespread use after World War II, laying the groundwork for modern medicine.

Along the way, livestock producers discovered that giving antibiotics to healthy pigs and chickens made them gain weight faster. Yet now scientists know that feeding antibiotics to healthy animals over time, especially in low doses, kills weak bacteria, allowing strains that can withstand the drugs to evolve and become dominant.

Bacteria that develop resistance to one antibiotic can often tolerate another, or several others. They can pass this trait not only to their offspring but to other microbes of different species.

Industrial-scale animal production is an ideal climate for breeding superbugs. It offers an environment in which bacteria can develop antibiotic resistance and spread it via human workers, animals, water, soil and air. Superbugs can travel on meat to stores - and into kitchens, where food safety missteps can make people sick.

Beware of Statins

Statins are now among the most widely prescribed drugs on the market with one in four Americans over 45 taking them, and are the number one profit-maker for the pharmaceutical industry, largely due to relentless and highly successful direct-to-consumer advertising campaigns.

In fact, a recent study assessing the effect of direct-to-consumer drug advertising concluded that TV ads for statins may be a driving factor of overdiagnosis of high cholesterol and overtreatment with the drugs.1

Statins are HMG-CoA reductase inhibitors, that is, they act by blocking the enzyme in your liver that is responsible for making cholesterol (HMG-CoA reductase).

The fact that statin drugs cause side effects is well established. A paper published in the ***American Journal of Cardiovascular Drugs*** cites nearly 900 studies on the adverse effects of HMG-CoA reductase inhibitors, also called statins, which run the gamut from muscle problems to increased cancer risk.

The biggest "sham" of all is that statin drugs, which millions are taking as a form of "preventive medicine" to protect their heart health, can have detrimental effects on your heart.

For example, a study published just last year in the journal *Atherosclerosis*, showed that statin use is associated with a 52 percent increased prevalence and extent of calcified coronary plaque compared to non-users. And coronary artery calcification is the *hallmark* of potentially lethal heart disease!

Now, researchers have uncovered yet another MAJOR problem associated with these drugs. One of the major benefits of exercise is the beneficial impact it has on your heart health, and exercise is a primary strategy to naturally maintain healthy cholesterol levels. Alas, if you take a statin drug, you're likely to forfeit any and all health benefits of your exercise.

Statins Can Undo the Benefits of Exercise

The study, published in the *Journal of the American College of Cardiology*4, discovered that statin use led to dramatically reduced fitness benefits from exercise, in some cases actually making the volunteer LESS fit than before!

The participants in the study included 37 overweight, sedentary men and women, all of whom had symptoms of metabolic problems, such as high blood pressure or excess abdominal fat. None of them had exercised regularly within the past 12 months, and most had slightly but not excessively elevated cholesterol levels.

Before the trial, muscle biopsies were taken from each participant to evaluate mitochondrial content, and their aerobic fitness was determined using treadmill testing. All participants were instructed to maintain their regular diet. The participants were then divided into two groups. One group was given a daily 40 mg dose of simvastatin (Zocor). The other group did not receive any medication. Both groups then began a supervised 12-week exercise program, walking or jogging on a treadmill for 45 minutes, five days a week. At the end of the three-month long trial, their aerobic fitness and muscles were retested. The results were astounding:

> On average, unmedicated volunteers improved their aerobic fitness by more than 10 percent. Mitochondrial content activity increased by 13 percent
>
> Volunteers taking 40mg of simvastatin improved their fitness by a mere 1.5 percent on average, and some had *reduced* their aerobic capacity at the end of the 12-week

fitness program. Mitochondrial content activity *decreased* by an average of 4.5 percent

According to senior study author John P. Thyfault, a professor of nutrition and exercise physiology at the University of Missouri:

"Low aerobic fitness is one of the best predictors of premature death. And if statins prevent people from raising their fitness through exercise, then that is a concern."

How Statins Might Undo Fitness Benefits and Make Your Heart Health Worse

The key to understanding why statins prevent your body from reaping the normal benefits from exercise lies in understanding what these drugs do to your mitochondria—the energy chamber of your cells, responsible for the utilization of energy for all metabolic functions.

The primary fuel for your mitochondria is Coenzyme Q10 (CoQ10), and one of the primary mechanisms of harm from statins in general appears to be related to CoQ10 depletion. This also explains why certain statin users in the featured trial ended up with *worse* aerobic fitness after a steady fitness regimen.

It's been known for many decades that exercise helps to build and strengthen your muscles, but more recent research has revealed that this is just the tip of the iceberg when it comes to the potential role exercise can play in your health. A 2011 review published in *Applied Physiology, Nutrition and Metabolism*6 pointed out that exercise induces changes in mitochondrial enzyme content and activity (which is what they tested in the featured study), which can increase your cellular energy production and in so doing decrease your risk of chronic disease.

The researchers stated:

"Increasing evidence now suggests that exercise can induce mitochondrial biogenesis in a wide range of tissues not normally associated with the metabolic demands of exercise. Perturbations [changes] in mitochondrial content and (or) function have been linked to a wide variety of diseases, in multiple tissues,

and exercise may serve as a potent approach by which to prevent and (or) treat these pathologies."

Increasing mitochondrial activity is incredibly important because free radicals, which are toxic byproducts of metabolism as well as exposures to chemicals, pollutants and other toxins, can overwhelm your body's defenses, leading to oxidative damage to cells and tissues that can destroy cellular proteins, lipids and DNA, as well as lead to the loss of mitochondrial function. In the long-term, irreversible damage in the mitochondria can occur, leading to:

- Lower threshold for physical exercise
- Impaired ability to utilize carbohydrates and fat for energy
- Insulin resistance
- Excessive weight gain
- Accelerated aging

If You're on a Statin Drug, You MUST Take CoQ10...

If you take a statin drug without supplementing with CoQ10—or ideally, the reduced form, called ubiquinol, which is far more effective—your health is at serious risk. CoQ10 is used by *every* cell in your body, but especially your heart cells. Cardiac muscle cells have up to 200 times more mitochondria, and hence 200 times higher CoQ10 requirements than skeletal muscle.

Now imagine if you start straining your heart with exercise and not counteracting the CoQ10 depletion caused by the drug... it's no wonder, really, that statin users couldn't improve their fitness levels! There simply wasn't enough mitochondrial fuel in their system. This is why supplementing with ubiquinol or CoQ10 is so critical when you're taking a statin drug. A recent study in the *European Journal of Pharmacology* showed that ubiquinol effectively rescued cells from the damage caused by the statin drug simvastatin, thereby protecting muscle cells from myopathies.

Premature aging is yet another side effect of statin drugs, and it's also a primary side effect of having too little CoQ10. Deficiency in this nutrient also accelerates DNA damage, and because CoQ10 is beneficial to heart health and muscle function this depletion leads to fatigue, muscle weakness, soreness and, ultimately, *heart failure...*

Again demonstrating the necessity of CoQ10 supplementation during statin therapy, a recent study evaluating the benefits of CoQ10 and selenium supplementation for patients with statin-associated myopathy found that, compared to those given a placebo, the treatment group experienced significantly less pain, decreased muscle weakness and cramps, and less fatigue.

"First and foremost, cholesterol is a vital component of every cell membrane on Earth. In other words, there is no life on Earth that can live without cholesterol. In fact, it is one of our best friends. We would not be here without it. No wonder lowering cholesterol too much increases one's risk of dying. Cholesterol is also a precursor to all of the steroid hormones. You cannot make estrogen, testosterone, cortisone, and a host of other vital hormones without cholesterol."

Beware the Health Hazards of Statin Drugs!

First, if you are a woman, it's critical for you to know that statins are classified as a "pregnancy Category X medication" meaning, *it causes serious birth defects,* and should NEVER be used if you're pregnant or planning a pregnancy. Last year, the US Food and Drug Administration9 (FDA) also announced it's considering additional warning labels for statin drugs. Among them are warnings that statins may increase your risk of:

- Liver damage
- Memory loss and confusion
- Type 2 diabetes
- Muscle weakness (for certain statins)

In all, statin drugs have been directly linked to over 300 side effect

https://www.npscript.com/dougcaporrino/coq10-100mg/AM0098PAR?skuID=AM0098

Women Beware

The issue of what kind of feminine hygiene products you use is rarely if ever discussed. Yet it's clearly an important topic for every woman out there.

Your skin is the largest organ in your body, and also the thinnest. Less than 1/10th of an inch separates your body from potential toxins. Worse yet, your skin is highly permeable — especially the skin around your vaginal area, not to mention inside the vagina itself.

This is why attention needs to be paid to the ingredients used in tampons and sanitary pads.

Most items that come in constant contact with your skin will end up in your bloodstream and distributed throughout your body. This is why I'm so fond of saying "don't put anything on your body that you wouldn't eat if you had to."

Putting chemicals on your skin may actually be worse than eating them. When you eat something, the enzymes in your saliva and stomach help to break it down and flush it out of your body.

However, when chemicals come in contact with your skin, they are absorbed straight into your bloodstream without filtering of any kind, going directly to your delicate organs. And once these chemicals find their way into your body, they tend to accumulate over time because you typically lack the necessary enzymes to break them down.

In my opinion, the realm of feminine hygiene can be likened to a "ticking time bomb." Because when you consider your exposure over the course of a lifetime, it really adds up; the average American woman uses up to 16,800 tampons in her lifetime — or as many as 24,360 if she's on estrogen replacement therapy.

And that's just tampons... Many women use countless sanitary pads in place of, or in addition to tampons. When this same 'average' woman has a baby, she may also use maternity and nursing pads.

What's Really in Those Sanitary Pads and Tampons?

Manufacturers of tampons and sanitary pads are not required to disclose the ingredients used because feminine hygiene products are considered "medical devices."

When an investigator called Procter & Gamble directly to find out what's in their Always Infinity pads, the only ingredients the service reps could give her were: foam and a patented ingredient called Infinicel2 — a highly absorbent material that can hold up to 10 times its weight.

In fact, according to her research, each conventional sanitary pad contains the equivalent of about four plastic bags! With everything we now know about the hazardous nature of plastic chemicals, this alone is cause for concern.

For example, plasticizing chemicals like BPA and BPS disrupt embryonic development and are linked to heart disease and cancer. Phthalates — which give paper tampon applicators that smooth feel and finish — are known to dysregulate gene expression, and DEHP may lead to multiple organ damage. Besides crude oil plastics, conventional sanitary pads can also contain a myriad of other potentially hazardous ingredients, such as odor neutralizers and fragrances. Synthetics and plastic also restrict the free flow of air and can trap heat and dampness, potentially promoting the growth of yeast and bacteria in your vaginal area.

The Price You Pay for 'Clean' White Tampons and Pads

Furthermore, to give tampons and pads that pristine, "clean" white look, the fibers used must be bleached. Chlorine is commonly used for this, which can create toxic dioxin and other disinfection-by-products (DBPs) such as triha-lom-ethane. Studies show that dioxin collects in your fatty tissues, and according to a draft report by the US Environmental

Protection Agency (EPA), dioxin a serious public health threat that has *no* "safe" level of exposure! Published reports show that even low or trace levels of dioxins may be linked to:

- Abnormal tissue growth in the abdomen and reproductive organs
- Abnormal cell growth throughout the body
- Immune system suppression
- Hormonal and endocrine system disruption

Meanwhile, the FDA's official stance regarding trace amounts of dioxins is that there are no expected health risks associated with trace amounts of dioxins in tampons... Naturally Savvy notes that 10 years ago, House Representative Carolyn Maloney introduced legislation that would have required research into the potential health risks of any ingredient used in feminine hygiene products, including endometriosis, cervical, ovary and breast cancers. Unfortunately, the legislation did not pass, and it does not appear that any such research has been done.

Could You Be Absorbing GMO's Via Your Tampons?

Investigators discovered a number of shocking details about the potential hazards posed by tampons and sanitary pads during research for a recent book called, *Label Lessons*, such as3:

- *Conventional tampons contain pesticides... Cotton crops make up just 2.4 percent of the world's land, but each year a whopping $2 billion is spent on pesticides to spray this one crop.*
- *Tampons and pads with odor neutralizers and other artificial fragrances are nothing short of a chemical soup laced with artificial colors, polyester, adhesives, polyethylene (PET), polypropylene, and propylene glycol (PEG), contaminants linked to hormone disruption, cancer, birth defects, dryness, and infertility.*
- *Conventional tampons most probably contain genetically modified organisms (GMOs). According the USDA, 94 percent of all the cotton planted in the US is genetically engineered.*

Beware of Toxic Shock Syndrome

It's important to remember that tampons can create a favorable environment for bacteria growth. Micro tears in the vaginal wall from tampons allow bacteria to enter and accumulate. One recognized risk from tampon use is Toxic Shock Syndrome (TSS), which may be caused by poisonous toxins from either Staphylococcus aureus (staph) or group A streptococcus (strep) bacteria. TSS can be a life-threatening condition.

To minimize your risk of this potentially life-threatening condition:

Avoid super absorbent tampons - choose the lowest absorbency rate to handle your flow	Never leave a tampon inserted overnight; use overnight pads instead	When inserting a tampon, be extremely careful not to scratch your vaginal lining (avoid plastic applicators)
Alternate the use of tampons with sanitary napkins or mini-pads during your period	Change tampons at least every 4-6 hours	Do not use a tampon between periods

Safer Alternatives

Many of today's feminine hygiene products are made primarily from rayon, vicose, and cellulose wood fluff pulp... *not* cotton — let alone organic cotton. Rayon and viscose present a potential danger in part because of their highly absorbent fibers. When used in tampons, these fibers can stick to your vaginal wall, and when you remove the tampon, the loosened fibers stay behind inside your body, thereby raising your risk of TSS.

Fortunately, there are safer alternatives, and since the FDA regulates tampon absorbency, all tampons on the market must meet the same absorption guidelines. According to NYU Medical Centre, 100 percent cotton tampons "consistently test under detectable levels for TSS toxins." Based on our research, we recommend the following brands of tampons and sanitary pads listed below.

- Natracare
- Diva Cup
- Seventh Generation Chlorine Free Organic Cotton Tampons
- Glad Rags Organic Pads
- Organic 100% Organic Cotton Tampons

Schools Can Be Danger Zones

Playgrounds, daycare centers and schools: every parent hopes these are safe places, where children can flourish and grow. Unfortunately, pesticides used in and near schools and playgrounds can make children an unintended 'frontline community,' exposing them to dangerous chemicals just when their developing brains and bodies are especially vulnerable.

Parents, communities and organizations around the country are finding ways to make schools safer for growing children. Progress includes pesticide use reduction in school buildings, buffer zones to protect children from spraying in nearby fields, and support for safer pest control methods in and near schools and playgrounds.

Contaminated Classrooms & Schoolyards

From the moment the morning school bell rings, children face a number of exposure risks. Pesticides can settle on desks, books, counters and walls. Children – and teachers – breathe contaminated air or touch contaminated surfaces, unknowingly exposing themselves to chemical residues that can remain in the school environment for days.

In rural areas, pesticides often drift into schoolyards from nearby fields

Of the 40 pesticides most commonly used in schools, 28 are probable or possible carcinogens, 26 have been shown to cause reproductive effects, 26 damage the nervous system, and 13 can cause birth defects.

In rural areas, pesticides often drift into schoolyards during and after applications on nearby fields. PAN's Drift Catcher has been used in communities across the country to document pesticides in or near school grounds.

- Schoolchildren in Strathmore, CA were exposed to pesticides sprayed in a neighboring field, feeling dizzy and falling sick in November, 2007.
- Seven children were hospitalized and a total of 11 people sickened in Kahuku, Hawaii in 2007, when fumes from an organophosphate insecticide drifted over the school from a nearby sod farm.
- In Florida, high school students used a PAN Drift Catcher to measure the pesticide endosulfan drifting into the school from nearby cabbage fields.

Pesticides, Playgrounds & Fields

Young children explore the world in very hands-on ways. Pesticides used to coat the wood of playground structures, keep landscaping tidy or fields weed-free can end up on small fingers - which often end up in small mouths. A young child's common hand-to-mouth behavior is well known to increase risk of pesticide exposure.

Communities across the country are confronting this risk to young children head-on, demanding safer play environments. In the Pacific Northwest, 17 cities have mandated pesticide free parks and playgrounds.

Pesticide use on playing fields has raised concerns among families and environmental health advocates nationwide. The National Coalition for Pesticide-Free Lawns notes that "the common, everyday practices used to maintain our children's playing fields are unintentionally and unnecessarily exposing them to carcinogens, and developmental toxins," and calls for a shift to organic turf management on playing fields across the country.

Communities are demanding safer play environments for children

Calls for Synthetic turf, touted by advocates as a "solution" to pesticides on playing fields, has actually raised other serious health concerns. The U.S. currently has about 3,500 synthetic playing fields made of various materials, including nylon and polyethylene, and about 800 are installed each year at schools, colleges, parks and stadiums, according to the industry's Synthetic Turf Council.

Pigment containing lead chromate is used in some surfaces to make the turf green and hold its color in sunlight, potentially exposing children and others using this turf to lead. Studies have also raised deep concerns about exposure to lead and other toxins from the crumb rubber infill used in many synthetic turf fields.

Creating Safer Spaces for Children

Thirty-six states now have school pesticide regulations, and pioneering districts across the country are developing least-toxic pest management approaches. A few examples:

- In 2005 Connecticut became the first U.S. state to ban use of synthetic weed killer pesticides around schools & daycare centers in grades K-8.
- In May 2010, New York Governor David Paterson signed the Child Safe Playing Fields Act into law, banning the cosmetic use of pesticides on playgrounds & sports fields at schools & daycare centers. The law also applies these protections to high schools.
- In California, the Healthy Schools Act mandates parent notification when pesticides are to be applied, and recommends least-toxic Integrated Pest Management for schools and daycares. Many local school districts have adopted health-protective policies, and several counties have enacted buffer zones, limiting aerial spraying of pesticides around schools, daycares and other sensitive sites. A new study examines the effectiveness of the Act in daycares.
- Dozens of municipalities in Canada, as well as the provinces of Quebec and Nova Scotia, have passed laws restricting "cosmetic" pesticide use for lawns & playgrounds. Ontario province recently banned use of 2,4-D in lawns & landscapes.

In 2009 EPA released a plan encouraging all public schools to adopt Integrated Pest Management by 2015. Experts calculate the approach could reduce school use of pesticides by at least 70%. Unfortunately, EPA's plan is a set of guidelines rather than a directive, and no funding to help schools switch from conventional pest management. The Schools Environmental Protection Act, introduced in 2009, would address these issues.

FDA approves first GMO Flu Vaccine containing Reprogrammed Insect Virus

A new vaccine for influenza has hit the market, and it is the first ever to contain genetically-modified (GM) proteins derived from insect cells. According to reports, the U.S. Food and Drug Administration (FDA) recently approved the vaccine, known as Flublok, which contains recombinant DNA technology and an insect virus known as baculovirus that is purported to help facilitate the more rapid production of vaccines.

According to Flublok's package insert, the vaccine is trivalent, which means it contains GM proteins from three different flu strains. The vaccine's manufacturer, Protein Sciences Corporation (PSC), explains that Flublok is produced by extracting cells from the fall armyworm, a type of caterpillar, and genetically altering them to produce large amounts of hemagglutinin, a flu virus protein that enables the flu virus itself to enter the body quickly.

So rather than have to produce vaccines the "traditional" way using egg cultures, vaccine manufacturers will now have the ability to rapidly produce large batches of flu virus protein using GMOs, which is sure to increase profits for the vaccine industry. But it is also sure to lead to all sorts of serious side effects, including the deadly nerve disease Guillain-Barre Syndrome (GSB), which is listed on the shot as a potential side effect.

"If Guillain-Barre Syndrome (GBS) has occurred within six weeks of receipt of a prior influenza vaccine, the decision to give Flublock should be based on careful consideration of the potential benefits and risks," explains a section of the vaccine's literature entitled "Warnings and Precautions." Other potential side effects include allergic reactions, respiratory infections, headaches, fatigue, altered immune-competence.

According to clinical data provided by PSC in Flublok's package insert, two study participants actually died during trials of the vaccine. But the company still insists Flublok is safe and effective, and that it is about 45 percent effective against all strains of influenza in circulation, rather than just one or two strains.

FDA also approves flu vaccine containing dog kidney cells

Back in November, the FDA also approved a new flu vaccine known as Flucel-vax that is actually made using dog kidney cells. A product of pharmaceutical giant Novartis, Flucelvax also does away with the egg cultures, and can similarly be produced much more rapidly than traditional flu vaccines, which means vaccine companies can have it ready and waiting should the federal government declare a pandemic.

Like Flublok, Flucelvax was made possible because of a $1 billion, taxpayer-funded grant given by the U.S. Department of Health and Human Services (HHS) to the vaccine industry back in 2006 to develop new manufacturing methods for vaccines. The ultimate goal is to be able to quickly manufacture hundreds of millions of vaccines for rapid distribution.

Meanwhile, there are reportedly two other GMO flu vaccines currently under development. One of them, which is being produced by Novavax, will utilize "bits of genetic material grown in caterpillar cells called 'virus-like particles' that mimic a flu virus," according to Reuters.

Keep Skin Young

You need to hydrate sufficiently by drinking lots of water and consuming fewer diuretics such as coffee. Assist your microbiome by washing your skin (especially your hands) regularly with soap and water, but do not use antibacterial soap. In addition to being toxic, it destroys your microbiome, which leaves you far more vulnerable to aggressive pathogens living on your skin. You also might want to think about putting a chlorine filter on your showerhead so as not to totally destroy those trillion beneficial bacteria living on your skin. Use a carnosine based supplement to slow down cell sene-scence and minimize protein degradation.

Use a full spectrum antioxidant. Make sure it contains resveratrol, which can reduce skin cancer tumors by 98% and stop the production of leukemia cells—in addition to slowing down the aging process. You'll also want your formula to contain OPC grape seed extract, which can revive declining capillary activity by up to 140% as well as repair varicose veins and prevent bruising.

Supplement with 4-10 mg of astaxanthin a day. Astaxanthin has not only been proven to protect your skin from the sun (it actually works as an internal sun screen) and reduce the signs of aging, but it has also been shown to profoundly suppress cancerous mutations in skin cells.

Supplement with systemic proteolytic enzymes and omega-3 fatty acids to reduce inflammation throughout the body, including the skin. Regular full body detoxing since toxins affect all organs, including your skin. Use a progesterone crème to balance out excess estrogen levels. Use a formula to free up bound testosterone. During and after menopause, you may want to use an all-natural estriol crème to rebalance declining estrogen levels.

Use an HGH supplement to help reestablish growth hormone levels in your body. Although not as powerful as HGH injections, these formulas can be quite effective (provided your pituitary is still functioning) and carry none of the downside of injections. The key ingredients in these formulas tend to be arginine (an essential amino acid) and GABA.

Collagen is a complex structural protein that maintains strength and flexibility throughout the body and especially the skin. Collagen levels in your skin decline as you age. Unfortunately, collagen molecules are so large and complex that they won't penetrate the outer layers of the skin so topical application is useless, and they don't readily pass through the walls of the digestive tract so supplementation is only marginally useful. Fortunately, you can now find supplements made from collagen peptides. The peptides are made by hydrolyzing (or breaking down) the large collagen molecules into smaller, low molecular weight molecules that can actually be absorbed and utilized by the body.

Hyaluronic acid (HA) is your skin's ultimate hydrating agent. It is primarily found in the papillary layer of your dermis, filling the spaces between the collagen fibers as part of a thick gel comprised of water, protein complexes, and hyaluronic acid. HA attracts and holds 1,000 times its own weight in water, which is what plumps your skin so that wrinkles and lines are less visible. This jelly-like complex transports essential nutrients from the bloodstream, via the capillaries in your skin. Supplementing with HA can boost moisture levels and minimize the appearance of fine lines and wrinkles

Mild facial scrubs help remove old dead skin cells from the surface of the skin making it easier for new cells to make their way up. This is especially important as you age, since the whole process of shedding old skin slows down. Versions are made for both men and women. And for goodness sake, stop furrowing your brow. Or as your mother always told you, "Stop making that face or it will become permanent."

What Are Zeolites?

A Zeolite is an alkaline mineral which is formed when lava and ash from volcanoes have a chemical reaction with the sodium of sea water. This reaction creates a cage like structure along with a negative charge which makes zeolite different than any other mineral on the planet today. The negative charge in the zeolite acts like a magnet in your body to attract the positively charged toxins and heavy metals, and trap them in the cage of the zeolite. Other products in the marketplace cause what is known as a "healing crisis" by re-exposing your body to all of the heavy metals and toxins when they pull them out of your body cells. Your body then is forced to re-filter them which comes with many negative side effects. With Zeolite's cage structure, it traps the toxins and heavy metals, so your body is not re-exposed to them. This is why Zeolite does not create negative reactions and provides concrete positive results in the detoxification process.

One of Nature's Miracles, "Zeolite", was created over thousands of years upon the earth and has been waiting for science to catch up, find it, discover its greatness and deliver it to mankind where it can do what it was created to do – improve people's lives and wellbeing. As science continues to expand our minds, we have learned the power of this amazing natural resource and as the leaders in this Zeolite field we are positioned to tell this story to the world.

In our everyday world today, toxins are everywhere! Evidence has been built about the effects of our toxic environment and what it has on our long term health. It is not good! Scientists have known for quite some time that pollution and pesticides can adversely affect human health, and mounting evidence now reveals far more serious, and even deadly connections between toxic exposure and a variety of diseases.

As toxins accumulate, they can have very negative effects on each and every system within our bodies. Our bodies are a precise machine that as these toxins build up over time, they can cause damage to neurological, immune, reproductive and endocrine systems. Some of these toxins can cause cancers, some are toxic to the brain and nervous system and some can even cause birth defects and diminish our body's overall immunity levels.

How do we counteract the long term build-up of Toxins in the body? Fortunately, there are natural compounds that do exist that can safely bind and remove these harmful toxins from the body. One group of such compounds includes some of the safest, most effective and natural detoxifying minerals known ----- They are comprised of what are called **ZEOLITE**

https://www.npscript.com/dougcaporrino/ultra-binder-universal-toxin-binder/QS0031PAR#undefined2

Beware of Most Green Cleaning Products

Commercial cleaning products, even "green" ones like Simple Green, clean faster than soap and water can. But this is because they contain small amounts of the most powerful grease-cutting class of chemicals known — glycol ethers.

Overexposure to glycol ethers can cause anemia, intoxication, and irritation of the eyes and nose.

In laboratory animals, low-level exposure to glycol ethers has caused birth defects and damage to sperm and testicles. The most commonly used glycol ether, 2-butoxyethanol, has been shown to cause liver cancer in animals.

"You are exposed to the glycol ethers when you inhale them as the cleaner is used ... Most glycol ethers can silently penetrate your skin and enter your bloodstream ... If that were not enough, the glycol ethers also go through natural rubber gloves and many types of plastic gloves without changing their appearance."

The typical American home contains 3-10 gallons of toxic materials, in the form of about 60 different kinds of hazardous household cleaning products. That's right, the very things you use to clean your house are actually the primary sources of toxins and indoor air pollution that Americans expose themselves to year after year. And many of the new "green" alternatives now being offered by major corporations are only green in name, as you will soon discover.

The Cost of Cleaning Your Home

Having a clean home should never cost you something as valuable as your health, but that's exactly what you're putting at risk when you use household cleaners and laundry detergents filled with many of the hazardous chemicals on the market today.

The problem is, when the chemicals in these common household products hit your skin and lungs, they go directly into your bloodstream, bypassing your body's natural defense system against toxins (the liver and kidneys).

This type of indoor pollution is particularly harmful to your health because just one application of a typical household cleaner can leave dangerous chemicals lingering in your indoor air for hours at a time. For people who spend a large amount of their day indoors, this can amount to a frequent chemical attacks on your lungs.

So, which Ingredients are Toxic?

Some of the ingredients in common household cleaners, laundry detergents, and even "green" cleaners that can create a toxic indoor environment include:

- Glycol ethers – Widespread use in paints, perfumes, soaps, cosmetics and foods. Cause fatigue, lethargy, nausea, and possible liver and kidney damage.
- Phthalates – Cause reproductive harm, endocrine disruption, cancer, organ damage.
- Perfumes – Cause headaches, sinus problems, asthma, may cause intoxication and "addiction."
- Phosphates - Manufacturers have reduced eliminated phosphates from laundry products, but no action has ever been taken on dishwasher detergents. Causes widespread environmental damage.

- Nonylphenol ethoxylates (NPEs), a common ingredient in laundry detergents and all-purpose cleaners, is banned in Europe, and known to be a potent endocrine disrupter. It's already thought to be the cause of male fish transforming into females in waterways around the world!
- Formaldehyde, found in spray and wick deodorizers, is a suspected carcinogen.
- Volatile organic compounds (VOCs), including 1,4-dichlorobenzene– Cause nose and throat irritation, dizziness, asthma.
- Petroleum solvents in floor cleaners may damage mucous membranes.
- Butyl cellosolve, found in many all-purpose and window cleaners. May damage your kidneys, bone marrow, liver and nervous system.
- Ammonia – irritating to the skin, eyes and lungs.
- Chlorine – irritating to the skin, eyes and lungs.
- Sodium Lauryl Sulfate - skin irritant, eye irritant, potential cancer causer.

Why "Green" Cleaning Products May NOT Necessarily be Green!

As more and more consumers are learning about the dangers of the products they use in their homes, "green" environmentally friendly options have sparked an industry revolution with a growing number of companies offering their own versions of eco-friendly cleaners. Some examples are Clorox Green Works Natural All-Purpose Cleaner, Simple Green, and Purex Natural Elements.

Unfortunately, the terms "green" and "natural" are nothing more than marketing terms; they're not rigid well accepted scientific terms, and they do not automatically equate to safety. This shouldn't come as a surprise to anyone who is even slightly familiar with how multinational corporations use marketing to manipulate the image of their products.

If you want a real treat, please pick up and read a highly recommended book on this subject called *Subliminal Persuasion: Influence & Marketing Secrets They Don't Want You To Know.* This book reveals the systematic techniques used to form opinions or ideologies, in ways that we never suspect. Multinational corporations, like big drug companies, are using these techniques all the time to deceive you.

Many large corporations are chomping at the bit, eager to reach into the wallets of modern, environmentally concerned consumers searching for green alternatives to the toxic stew of chemicals found in conventional cleaning products. "Green" cleaning products are a growing niche market, with green cleaning product U.S. sales totaling $100 million in 2010.

But most "green" cleaning products like Simple Green are still loaded with glycol ethers, which are anything but good for your health when inhaled or when they touch your skin. Folks, the simple truth is that if a substance cuts through grease and dirt any faster than soap and water, then there are chemicals in there that most likely aren't very good for your health.

Why Glycol Ethers are BAD for You

Glycol ether is a generic term for over thirty solvents derived from crude oil, all with different properties, which are used in applications ranging from paints to inks to degreasing agents and cleaning products. Generally speaking, glycol ethers are hazardous when they get on your skin or when they get in your lungs. This is especially true with cleaning products, which are often applied indoors and without proper ventilation.

Reading the Labels Won't Always Help

I always advocate reading the labels on the foods and cleaning products you buy, but in the case of household cleaners even the most meticulous eye for labels won't get you very far.

Why?

Because many of the most dangerous chemicals will not even be on the label. The manufacturers have conveniently lobbied the government to exempt them from this requirement and can omit any ingredient that is considered a secret formula from its label. Many of these non-disclosed ingredients are actually toxic and carcinogenic.

Household goods are still very much an unregulated market. And, cleaning product manufacturers — even those that claim to be "green" — are not required by law to disclose all of their ingredients on their labels. So, while it's still better to read the label than not, be aware that a lack of ingredient on a label doesn't necessarily mean it's not in the product!

The Importance of Combating Chronic Inflammation

Inflammation is a normal and beneficial process that occurs when your body's white blood cells and chemicals protect you from foreign invaders like bacteria and viruses.

You actually need *some* level of inflammation in your body to stay healthy, however it's also possible, and increasingly common, for the inflammatory response to get out of hand. If your immune system mistakenly triggers an inflammatory response when no threat is present, it can lead to excess inflammation in your body, a condition linked to asthma, allergies, autoimmune disease, heart disease, cancer and other diseases, depending on which organs the inflammation is impacting.

Unfortunately, chronic inflammation typically will not produce symptoms until actual loss of function occurs somewhere. This is because chronic inflammation is low-grade and systemic, often silently damaging your tissues over an extended period of time. This process can go on *for years* without you noticing, until a disease suddenly sets in.

Diet accounts for about 80 percent of the health benefits you reap from a healthful lifestyle, and keeping inflammation in check is a major part of these benefits. It's important to realize that dietary components can either *trigger* or *prevent* inflammation from taking root in your body. For example, whereas trans fats and sugar, particularly fructose, will increase inflammation, eating healthy fats such as animal-based omega-3 fats found in krill oil, or the essential fatty acid gamma linolenic acid (GLA) will help to reduce them.

If you have not already addressed your diet, this would be the best place to start, regardless of whether you're experiencing symptoms of chronic inflammation or not.

But diet is not the only component that will have a profound impact on your health and longevity. It's really about addressing your total lifestyle. Here are a few of the components I believe have the greatest impact. All of these components affect chronic inflammation, but they also have other health ramifications.

Optimizing Your Insulin Levels is Paramount for a Long, Healthy Life

Having high insulin levels is a surefire way to speed up your aging process. If there's a single marker for lifespan, it would be insulin, specifically insulin sensitivity. Insulin resistance is the basis of virtually ALL of chronic diseases of aging, and one of the primary reasons for this is because it promotes chronic inflammation throughout your body.

Unfortunately, many health care practitioners are still ignorant of the profound influence that insulin has on health. Please understand that a firm appreciation of insulin's role is one of the most important things you can do to optimize your health and outlive the naysayers. The two most important elements for normalizing your insulin levels and avoiding insulin resistance are:

- Avoiding sugar/fructose and grains (remember that beverages play a paramount role here, as high fructose corn syrup from soda is one of the primary sources of calories in the US)
- Regular exercise

Argentina link health problems to agrochemicals

American biotechnology has turned Argentina into the world's third-largest soy producer, but the chemicals powering the boom aren't confined to soy and cotton and corn fields. The Associated Press documented dozens of cases where these poisons are used in ways specifically banned by existing law.

Now doctors are warning that uncontrolled pesticide use could be the cause of growing health problems among the 12 million people who live in the South American nation's vast farm belt.

In Santa Fe province, the heart of Argentina's soy industry, cancer rates are two times to four times higher than the national average. In Chaco, the nation's poorest province, children became four times more likely to be born with devastating birth defects in the decade since biotechnology dramatically expanded industrial agriculture.

"The change in how agriculture is produced has brought, frankly, a change in the profile of diseases," says Dr. Medardo Avila Vazquez, a pediatrician who co-founded Doctors of Fumigated Towns. "We've gone from a pretty healthy population to one with a high rate of cancer, birth defects, and illnesses seldom seen before."

Once known for its grass-fed beef, Argentina has undergone a remarkable transformation since 1996, when the St. Louis-based Monsanto

Company marketed a promising new model of higher crop yields and fewer pesticides through its patented seeds and chemicals.

Today, all of Argentina's soy and nearly all its corn, wheat and cotton are genetically modified. Soy farming tripled to 47 million acres (19 million hectares), and just like in the U.S., cattle are now fattened in feedlots on corn and soy.

But as weeds and insects became resistant, farmers increased the chemical burden eightfold, from 9 million gallons in 1990 to more than 84 million gallons today. Overall, Argentine farmers apply an estimated 4.3 pounds of agrochemical concentrate per acre, more than twice what U.S. farmers use, according to an AP analysis of government and pesticide industry data.

Monsanto's "Roundup" pesticides use glyphosate, one of the world's most widely applied and least toxic weed killers. The U.S. Environmental Protection Agency and many others have declared it to be safe if applied properly. In May, the EPA even increased allowable glyphosate residues on foods.

Despite the wholesale adoption of Monsanto's model, safety rules vary.

Some of Argentina's 23 provinces ban spraying within (1.9 miles) of populated areas; others say farmers can spray as close as (55 yards). About one-third set no limits, and rule-breakers are very rarely punished.

A federal law requires toxic chemical applicators to suspend activities that threaten public health, "even when the link has not been scientifically proven," and "no matter the costs or consequences," but it has never been applied to farming, the Auditor General found last year.

In response to soaring complaints, President Cristina Fernandez ordered a commission in 2009 to study the impact of agrochemical spraying on human health. Its initial report called for "systematic controls over concentrations of herbicides and their compounds ... such as exhaustive laboratory and field studies involving formulations containing glyphosate as well as its interactions with other agrochemicals as they are actually used in our country."

But the commission hasn't met since 2010, the auditor general found.

In a written statement, Monsanto spokesman Thomas Helscher said the company "does not condone the misuse of pesticides or the violation of any pesticide law, regulation, or court ruling."

"Monsanto takes the stewardship of products seriously and we communicate regularly with our customers regarding proper use of our products," Helscher said.

Argentina was among the earliest adopters of the "no-till" method U.S. agribusinesses promoted. Instead of turning the topsoil, spraying pesticides, and then waiting until the poison dissipates before planting, farmers sow seeds and spray afterward without harming "Roundup Ready" crops genetically modified to tolerate specific poisons. Farmers can now harvest multiple crops each year on land that wasn't profitable before.

But pests quickly develop resistance to the same chemicals applied to identical crops on a vast scale, forcing farmers to mix in more toxic poisons, such as 2,4,D, used in "Agent Orange" to defoliate Vietnam's jungles. Some Argentine regulators called for labels warning that these mixtures should be limited to "farm areas far from homes and population centers," but they were ignored, the auditor found.

"Glyphosate is even less toxic than the repellent you put on your children's skin," said Pablo Vaquero, Monsanto's spokesman in Buenos Aires. "That said, there has to be a responsible and good use of these products, because in no way would you put repellent in the mouths of children and no environmental applicator should spray fields with a tractor or a crop-duster without taking into account the environmental conditions and threats that stem from the use of the product."

Teachers in Entre Rios began to file police complaints this year. They said sprayers failed to respect (55-yard) limits at 18 schools, dousing 11 during class.

In Santa Fe, Druetta also filed complaints, saying her students fainted when pesticides drifted into their classrooms and that her school lacks safe drinking water.

A house-to-house epidemiological study of 65,000 people in Santa Fe, at the National University of Rosario, found cancer rates two times to four times higher than the national average, as well as thyroid disorders, respiratory illnesses and other afflictions seldom seen before.

"It could be linked to agrochemicals.. "They do all sorts of analysis for toxicity of the first ingredient, but they have never studied the interactions between all the chemicals they're applying."

Hospital records show birth defects quadrupled in Chaco, from 19.1 per 10,000 to 85.3 per 10,000, in the decade after genetically modified crops were approved. A medical team then surveyed 2,051 people in six towns, finding more disease wherever people are surrounded by farms.

In the farming village of Avia Terai, 31 percent said a family member had cancer, compared with 3 percent in the ranching village of Charadai. They also documented children with malformed skulls, exposed spinal cords, blindness and deafness, neurological damage and strange skin problems.

Japan Halts HPV Shot for Girls over Safety Issues

Japanese health officials have recorded nearly 2,000 adverse reactions—hundreds of them serious—in girls who got a dangerous U.S. government-backed cervical cancer vaccine that's also been linked to thousands of debilitating side effects in this country.

The alarming reports have led Japan's government to act, suspending recommendation for the controversial vaccine which is billed as a miracle shot that can prevent certain strains of cervical cancer caused by Human Papillomavirus (HPV). The U.S. government has taken the opposite approach amid equally alarming cases of serious side effects. Not only does the Obama administration continue recommending the vaccine (Gardasil), it spends large sums of taxpayer dollars promoting it and works hard to keep details involving its dangers secret.

Judicial Watch has reported extensively on this and uncovered droves of government records that show Gardasil has been linked to seizures, blindness, paralysis, speech problems, pancreatitis, short-term memory loss and dozens of deaths. Incredibly, the Food and Drug Administration (FDA) fast-tracked Gardasil's approval and the Centers for Disease Control and Prevention (CDC) recommends it for girls starting at age 9. JW has investigated the Gardasil scandal since 2007 and had to sue for the records in the face of Obama administration stonewalling.

In Japan Gardasil's disturbing side effects have been taken seriously by the Japanese Ministry of Health, Labor and Welfare (JMHLW), which has issued a warning to local governments that the HPV vaccine should not be recommended amid safety concerns. The information comes from a report issued this month by a Japanese internist and cardiologist, who reveals that the manufacturers' own documents indicate the HPV vaccine may induce seizures and/or brain damage. Besides Gardasil, he also reviewed another brand called Cervarix.

Taking the U.S. government's lead, the Japanese government pushed the vaccine countrywide, allocating 15 billion yen ($187.5 million) for "urgent HPV Vaccination programs" for girls ages 11 to 14. Officials visited junior high schools to advocate the effectiveness of the vaccine and persuade girls to get it. Municipal offices sent letters to families of girls in the targeted age group and the government stressed that the expensive vaccine (48,000 yen, $600, for three shots) would be free for only two years.

But health officials were taken aback with the high number of side effects reported to Japan's Vaccine Adverse Reactions Review Committee. Since the government began offering girls HPV shots, 1,968 adverse events were reported, including 358 that were evaluated as serious. Parents began calling the country's health minister and furnishing videos in which girls who had received the HPV vaccine suffered from walking disturbances, body tics and seizures. In other cases many girls injected with the vaccine fell to the floor, injuring their head or face and some fracturing their jaw or teeth.

In mid-June Japan's Vaccine Adverse Reactions Review Committee suspended recommendation for HPV vaccination. That same day health officials sent formal notifications to local governments saying that HPV vaccination should not be recommended until safety concerns got addressed by the appropriate agencies. American health officials, on the other hand, continue promoting it. In fact, weeks after Japan took action, the Obama administration dedicated $1.2 million to "increase HPV vaccine uptake in low income ethnic minority populations".

Why Fermented Foods Improve Health?

Fermented foods are foods that have been through a process of lactofermentation in which natural bacteria feed on the sugar and starch in the food creating lactic acid. This process preserves the food, and creates beneficial enzymes, b-vitamins, Omega-3 fatty acids, and various strains of probiotics.

Natural fermentation of foods has also been shown to preserve nutrients in food and break the food down to a more digestible form. This, along with the bevy of probiotics created during the fermentation process, could explain the link between consumption of fermented foods and improved digestion.

Cultures around the world have been eating fermented foods for years, from Sauerkraut in Germany to Kimchi in Korea and everywhere in between. Studies have even shown the link between probiotic rich foods and overall health. Sadly, with the advances in technology and food preparation, these time-honored traditional foods have been largely lost in our society.

Where Have All the Fermented Foods Gone?

The amount of probiotics and enzymes available in the average diet has declined sharply over the last few decades as pasteurized milk has replaced raw, pasteurized yogurt has replaced homemade, vinegar based pickles and sauerkraut have replaced traditional lacto-fermented versions… the list goes on.

Even the much dreaded grains were safer to eat in earlier times since their preparation included soaking, sprouting and fermenting, which largely reduces the anti-nutrient content and makes them less harmful (I still didn't say good!).

Instead of the nutrient rich foods full of enzymes and probiotics that our grandparents probably ate, the average diet today consists mainly of sugar laden, lab created dead foods.

Why Eat Fermented Foods?

Besides the fact that they taste great and really grow on you, there are several great reasons to start making and eating fermented foods:

1. **Probiotics**- Eating fermented foods and drinking fermented drinks like Kefir and Kombucha will introduce beneficial bacteria into your digestive system and help the balance of bacteria in your digestive system. Probiotics have also been shown to help slow or reverse some diseases, improve bowel health, aid digestion, and improve immunity!
2. **Absorb Food Better**- Having the proper balance of gut bacteria and enough digestive enzymes helps you absorb more of the nutrients in the foods you eat. Pair this with your healthy real food diet, and you will absorb many more nutrients from the foods you eat. You won't need as many supplements and vitamins, and you'll be absorbing more of the live nutrients in your foods.
3. **Budget Friendly**- Incorporating healthy foods into your diet can get expensive, but not so with fermented foods. You can make your own whey at home for a couple of dollars, and using that and sea salt, ferment many foods very inexpensively. Drinks like Water Kefir and Kombucha can be made at home also and cost only pennies per serving. Adding these things to your diet can also cut down on the number of supplements you need, helping the budget further.

4. **Preserves Food Easily**- Homemade salsa only lasts a few days in the fridge- Fermented homemade salsa lasts months! The same goes for sauerkraut, pickles, beets and other garden foods. Lacto-fermentation allows you to store these foods for longer periods of time without losing the nutrients like you would with traditional canning.

Stevia: Why it's Good for You and Which Ones to Buy

Origins

The stevia plant is part of the large sunflower family and native to subtropical parts of South and Central America, Mexico, and the US states Arizona, New Mexico and Texas. The Guarani people were historically nomadic and are now known to Paraguay, parts of Argentina, Brazil, Uruguay and Bolivia. The Guarani are said to have used the "candy leaf" for more than 1500 years.

This nation of people has used the herb for sweetening *mate*, a common tea drink, as well as a refreshing treat just chewing the leaf. But they've also known it to be medicinal, and to this day herbal medicine in Paraguay and Brazil uses stevia to treat illness and promote health.

Modern Use

Notably, Japan has also been using the plant leaf and one of its extracts, sativoside, for many decades. In fact, after years of rigorous testing to ensure the plant's safety, stevia now dominates 40% of all table and food additive sweeteners in the Land of the Rising Sun.

Additionally, many outside of the US have long since found that stevia can help to protect the gums and teeth, making it suitable for use in toothpastes and mouthwashes.

In the US, however, there has been controversy. Despite the plant's 1500+ year track record of approval, the FDA banned its import in 1991 calling the sweet leaf an unsafe food additive. There was and is a common assertion that the FDA's original rejection was not in the interest of public health, but Monsanto's booming line of artificial sweeteners. Whatever the case, the ban was greatly contested and by 1994, lifted. From there, sellers had to position and market stevia as a nutritional supplement, marginalizing the product to health-buffs and possibly preventing a mass exodus of calorie-counting buyers from the synthetic to the leaf.

Fifteen years later the FDA gave the nod, not to the use of the whole plant but to extraction of so-named "active constituents." Today, the whole stevia plant is still considered a supplement and *cannot* be used as a food additive. But as of 2009, instead of the whole leaf, the FDA has approved the use of "stevia-based" sweeteners.

This makes the products patentable. A plant cannot be patented and owned; but a process of extraction and the resulting product can be, and this makes for much better profits to the manufacturer. Thus, Coca Cola and PepsiCo grabbed their corner of the sugarless market via their products *Truvia* and *PureVia*, respectively. These are NOT recommended since their chemical makeup has been altered to make it patentable.

Therapeutic Value of Stevia

According to a report from the Pakistan Agricultural Research Council:

In addition to being a sweetener, stevia is considered (in Brazilian herbal medicine) to be hypoglycemic, hypotensive, diuretic, cardiotonic and tonic. *The leaf is used for* diabetes, *obesity, cavities, hypertension, fatigue,* depression, *sweet cravings, and infections. The leaf is employed in traditional medical systems in Paraguay and Brazil.*

Sweet Leaf and Blood Sugar

Numerous animal and human studies from around the world have demonstrated that stevia is safe. One of the hottest questions in the scientific community now is whether or not the leaf also has the power to keep blood sugar levels under control.

In a 2011 animal study, researchers fed diabetes-induced rats stevia for 10 days and compared the results to a placebo group. The blood glucose level of the stevia group showed "delayed but significant decrease," yet, unlike the conventional drugs, it did *not* cause hypoglycemia. This is GOOD.

The herb has been shown to nourish the pancreas and encourage more insulin production, perhaps lending to the increase of insulin and insulin sensitivity. But these results are still inconclusive. Concerning its efficacy in improving the type 2 diabetic condition, there have been mixed results. Some have found that people with type 2 diabetes experience significantly lowered blood sugar after consuming stevia; whereas others have shown little to no difference. Nevertheless, people in Brazil and Paraguay have been using the herb to prevent and treat the condition. No doubt, further clinical and epidemiological studies need to be done.

Importantly for type 2 diabetics and others looking to swat out sugar, **the natural sweet leaf has a glycemic load of 0, which means it does not raise blood sugar or cause an insulin spike.**

Improves Hypertension, Heals Wounds and More

Research over the years has also shown that stevia may help to lower high blood pressure. Some skincare products have incorporated the ingredient as a skin tightener and to improve complexion. Since the first millennium stevia has been applied to wounds for its antibacterial cleansing powers and to assist in healing. Some have even claimed results applying it to flare-ups of eczema, psoriasis and dermatitis. If you have one of these on your scalp, for instance, proponents say try adding a little whole leaf stevia extract to your shampoo. It may burn a wee bit at first, but the discomfort should quickly subside and you may see an overall reduction in inflammation, redness, itching and flaking.

Potential Counterfeits & What to Buy

It's likely that stevia's health benefits are real but mild and varied, but there is no scientific argument against its benefits as a sugar replacement, nor its safety as a food additive. Yet, the FDA has done a strange thing:

- They've declared as potentially unsafe a leaf that has been apparently safely used for a screamingly long time;
- put the stamp-of-approval on toxic chemical artificial sweeteners that are now demonstrated to cause cancer and a slew of mild and severe chronic illnesses including obesity and diabetes.

To make the sweetener, rebiana is pulled out from stevia's synergistic body of plant chemicals and used solely for its strength as a sweetener. We've thoroughly researched and observed the safety of the whole leaf, but how do we know that rebaudioside A is, by itself, completely safe over the long haul?

Answer: we don't.

It could be, but as of yet we don't have enough experience or long-term studies to be sure. Without the remaining agents of the plant our bodies are likely to respond differently. Even if nature fully provided all we need to properly digest and make use of the plant, by throwing out everything but the sweet we could find ourselves snagged in a health risk, yet again.

So, my recommendation is to stick to the whole leaf at least until we know more. Whole leaf stevia can have a strong aftertaste, but this is largely a result of the method of processing. Try out different brands till you find the one you like best.

Stevia can be enjoyed in beverages, salad dressings, cooking, baking and more.

4 Dirty Secrets of the Seafood Industry

The fishing industry is isolated from public view, so you rarely see the long, dirty road your seafood takes from ocean to plate.

Oceans cover 70 percent of the world's surface and host such a huge variety of life that new species are discovered all the time, and a billion people on earth depend on the oceans for their primary source of animal protein—fish. But supplying them, along with seafood-loving Americans, Europeans, and residents of increasingly wealthy Asian nations, is taking a huge toll, not just on our oceans, but on our health, too.

The seafood industry has the benefit of operating in the middle of the ocean, far, far outside the public scrutiny that has revealed the unhealthy and destructive practices of land-based factory farms and other forms of agriculture. As a result, the industry has been able to hide some of its worst tactics for satisfying our insatiable demand for omega-3s.

Here are some of the surprising facts they revealed:

#1: Just 1 percent of the world's fishing ships catch up to 50 percent of the world's fish. As with land-based agriculture, just a handful of major fishing corporations control a huge percentage of the seafood that's caught all over the world. And those big companies favor big, destructive equipment. Massive "supertrawlers," as they're sometimes called, drag huge nets—some of which are so huge they could hold twelve

747 airplanes—that stir up the sea floor and flush fish out of their hiding spots. The largest of these gargantuan ships, the Atlantic Dawn, can haul in 300 tons of fish *every day*—that's enough to feed 18 million people one fish dinner daily. The ship also has an onboard fish-processing facility that flash-freezes its haul so the fish are ready to ship to restaurants and grocers as soon as Atlantic Dawn pulls into port at the end of its months-long fishing trips.

Eat local. The other 99 percent of the world's fishing fleet is made up of small and artisanal fishermen who are more conscientious about maintaining healthy fisheries. While there are small fishermen who use trawls and other destructive fishing methods, buying local fish—like buying local meat—allows you to grill your meal about where the fish comes from and how it was caught.

#2: Our love of shrimp may very well be killing the Gulf of Mexico. Roughly a third of all fish pulled out of the oceans are considered by catch, non-target species that find themselves in nets or on hooks meant for other fish. Those fish get tossed back into the ocean, dead or dying, despite the fact that some bycatch species, such as cod, are commercially valuable. Shrimp trawling is one of the biggest offenders: Shrimp trawlers in the Gulf of Mexico pull up between three and five pounds of bycatch for every pound of shrimp. Picture three to five pounds of other sea creatures on the table with you while you're eating shrimp it's pretty sad.

Furthermore, those trawlers, which drag their nets along sea floors looking for shrimp that live in the mud, are notorious for catching and killing sea turtles, six species of which inhabit the Gulf. All six have been classified as threatened or endangered and are protected under the Endangered Species Act. However, shrimping companies have lobbied for concessions that allow them to kill the turtles.

Don't eat shrimp. There's no way to eat shrimp and feel good about it. Farmed shrimp, the alternative to wild, may not kill sea turtles but it's filthy. If you're eating farmed shrimp, it was grown in a shallow pond in the coastal zone of some hot tropical country, packed with thousands of other shrimp in muddy water where fecal matter piles up. The fish are dosed with chemicals to keep healthy while they live in these conditions. It's like a chicken farm under water. There are, however, other choices when it comes to sustainable shrimp farming. This website gives you a good look at what companies are doing their best: https://www.seafoodwatch.org/seafood-recommendations/groups/shrimp.

#3: Tuna processors are processing out all the good stuff. It's not just fishing methods that are unhealthy. The healthfulness of canned seafood, particularly tuna, takes a hit when the seafood industry gets its hands on it.

Here's the standard method that a whole tuna gets from the ocean to a can:

First, a frozen tuna gets defrosted and cooked under high heat and pressure in a huge oven. During that process, all the fats and oils drip out from the tuna and get collected to be resold as additives for animal feed or for other uses, for instance, fish oil supplements. Once it's cooked, workers strip the meat off the bone and send it into packaging machinery where it's placed into cans. At that point, the meat is fairly dried out because it's already been roasted and is devoid of any juices and fat. If processors simply canned that, it would scorch and stick to the can. So, processors add a solution of soy-based vegetable broth and pyrophosphate, a food additive. But those do more than just protect the meat from scorching. The broth contains hydrolyzed vegetable protein, which binds to the pyrophosphate to create something that looks like tuna and therefore adds bulk and protein to the tuna meat that's already there, so it looks like you're getting a full 5 ounces of tuna, when in reality you're getting just 3.5 ounces of tuna and 1.5 ounces of water and additives. Finally, a lid is put on the can and the tuna is cooked a second time, for roughly an hour, to sterilize it.

All this "makes the cost of a tuna can cheaper," but a breakdown of the three biggest supermarket brands shows just how much that cheap tuna is providing. (The figures below are based on 2-ounce servings of solid white albacore tuna in water.) Bumble Bee: 13 g protein; 100 mg omega-3s Chicken of the Sea: 13 g protein; 150 mg omega-3s Starkist: 12 g protein; 110 mg omega-3s

Eat healthier tuna. Compare those figures with the three leading sustainable brands of tuna which can a full 5 ounces of raw tuna meat with a little salt and nothing more, then cooking it just once via pressure cooking to sterilize the can and the contents. They capture the drippings that the conventional method loses during the first cooking phase in the can, and that becomes our liquid,". It also contains all the good omega-3s that make seafood so healthy (and more protein, which comes from fish, not from food additives). American Tuna: 14 g protein; 2,667 to 3,333 mg omega-3s Vital Choice: 16 g protein; 1,653 mg omega-3s Wild Planet: 16 g protein; 1,340 mg omega-3s.

As an added bonus, all of those brands catch younger tuna, which have lower levels of mercury than the larger fish favored by national brands, using much less environmentally damaging pole-and-line fishing methods.

#4: The seafood you *think* you're eating is probably not what you're eating. Increasing attention has been paid in recent years to the very serious issue of "seafood fraud," in which distributors, retailers, or restaurateurs sell you mislabeled fish. For instance, labeling a fish as "tuna" when it is in fact eel. Sometimes the deception is intentional. Illegal fishermen, who catch between 13 and 31 percent of the world's seafood, often try to pass off their catch as something that came from a legitimate fishery, despite the fact that it may have been caught in violation of international quotas or treaties, Sometimes the restaurateur is buying from a supplier who may or may not be reliable," once a fish is filleted is becomes easy to pass off as anything an unscrupulous salesman says it is.

The result? You get environmentally damaging and potentially dangerous fish. Oceana has conducted studies in major cities across the U.S. and found that a third of all fish sold in grocery stores and restaurants—sushi joints are particularly prone to fraud, they found—is mislabeled. Their DNA testers found that fish labeled red snapper, an overfished species subject to tight regulation, was actually tilefish, which is known to harbor dangerously high mercury levels. Fish passed off as expensive tuna varieties in U.S. sushi restaurants were actually escolar, "a fish with such a nasty reputation for its gastrointestinal effects it's been dubbed the Ex-Lax fish," Escolar is even banned in Japan.

America could establish traceability and labeling requirements, which would go a long way toward eliminating fraud. However, such labeling is unlikely anytime soon. Whole Foods, has established a thorough seafood traceability program at its stores, as have a few other big-chain grocers. Alternatively, you can look for local fishermen who sell their local catch.

Fish You Should Never Eat

Steer clear of this seafood that's bad for you and the environment

One fish, two fish, bad-for-you-fish. Yes fish, no fish, red fish…OK fish? Our oceans have become so depleted of wild fish stocks, and so polluted with industrial contaminants, that trying to figure out the fish that are both safe and sustainable can make your head spin. "Good fish" lists can change year after year, because stocks rebound or get depleted every few years, but there are some fish that, no matter what, you can always decline.

The nonprofit Food and Water Watch looked at all the varieties of fish out there, how they were harvested, how certain species are farmed, and levels of toxic contaminants like mercury or PCBs in the fish, as well as how heavily local fishermen relied upon fisheries for their economic survival. These are the 12 fish, they determined, that all of us should avoid, no matter what.

Imported Catfish Why It's Bad: Nearly 90% of the catfish imported to the US comes from Vietnam, where use of antibiotics that are banned in the U.S. is widespread. Furthermore, the two varieties of Vietnamese catfish sold in the US, Swai and Basa, aren't technically considered catfish by the federal government and therefore aren't held to the same inspection rules that other imported catfish are.

Stick with domestic, farm-raised catfish,. It's responsibly farmed and plentiful, making it one of the best fish you can eat. As long as it's organic. Or, try Asian carp, an invasive species with a similar taste to catfish that's out-competing wild catfish and endangering the Great Lakes ecosystem.

Why It's Bad: Caviar from beluga and wild-caught sturgeon are susceptible to overfishing, according to the Food and Water Watch report, but the species are also being threatened by an increase in dam building that pollutes the water in which they live. All forms of caviar come from fish that take a long time to mature, which means that it takes a while for populations to rebound.

If you really love caviar, opt for fish eggs from American Lake Sturgeon or American Hackleback/Shovelnose Sturgeon caviar from the Mississippi River system.

Atlantic Cod Why It's Bad: This one was difficult to add to the "dirty dozen list,", because it is so vital to the economic health of New England fishermen. "However, chronic mismanagement by the National Marine Fisheries Service and low stock status made it very difficult to recommend,". Atlantic cod stocks collapsed in the mid-1990s and are in such disarray that the species is now listed as one step above endangered on the International Union for Conservation of Nature's Red List of Threatened Species.

The good news, if you love fish 'n' chips (which is nearly always made with cod), is that Pacific cod stocks are still strong and are one of Food and Water Watch's best fish picks.

American Eel Why It's Bad: Also called yellow or silver eel, this fish, which frequently winds up in sushi dishes, made its way onto the list because it's highly contaminated with PCBs and mercury. The fisheries are also suffering from some pollution and overharvesting.

If you like the taste of eel, opt for Atlantic- or Pacific-caught squid instead.

Imported Shrimp Why It's Bad: Imported shrimp actually holds the designation of being the dirtiest of the Dirty Dozen, and it's hard to avoid, as 90% of shrimp sold in the U.S. is imported. "Imported farmed shrimp comes with a whole bevy of contaminants: antibiotics, residues from chemicals used to clean pens, filth like mouse hair, rat hair, and pieces of insects,". "And I didn't even mention things like E. coli that have been detected in imported shrimp." Part of this has to do with the fact that less than 2% of ALL imported seafood (shrimp, crab, catfish, or others) gets inspected before its sold, which is why it's that much more important to buy domestic seafood. Still need convincing?

Look for domestic shrimp. Seventy percent of domestic shrimp comes from the Gulf of Mexico, which relies heavily on shrimp for economic reasons. Pink shrimp from Oregon are another good choice; the fisheries there are certified under the stringent Marine Stewardship Council guidelines.

Atlantic Flatfish Why It's Bad: This group of fish includes flounder, sole, and halibut that are caught off the Atlantic coast. They found their way onto the list because of heavy contamination and overfishing that dates back to the 1800s. According to Food and Water Watch, populations of these fish are as low as 1% of what's necessary to be considered sustainable for long-term fishing. Pacific halibut seems to be doing well, but the group also recommends replacing these fish with other mild-flavored white-fleshed fish, such as domestically farmed catfish or tilapia.

Atlantic Salmon (both wild-caught and farmed) Why It's Bad: It's actually illegal to capture wild Atlantic salmon because the fish stocks are so low, and they're low, in part, because of farmed salmon. Salmon farming is very polluting: Thousands of fish are crammed into pens, which leads to the growth of diseases and parasites that require antibiotics and pesticides. Often, the fish escape and compete with native fish for food, leading to declines in native populations. Adding to our salmon woes, the U.S. Food and Drug Administration is moving forward with approving genetically engineered salmon to be sold, unlabeled, to unsuspecting seafood lovers. That salmon would be farmed off the coast of Panama, and it's unclear how it would be labeled. Currently, all fish labeled "Atlantic salmon" come from fish farms.

Opt for wild Alaskan salmon now, and in the event that GE salmon is officially approved.

Imported King Crab Why It's Bad: The biggest problem with imported crab is that most of it comes from Russia, where limits on fish harvests aren't strongly enforced. But this crab also suffers from something of an identity crisis. Imported king crab is often misnamed Alaskan king crab, because most people think that's name of the crab.

Alaskan king crab is a completely separate animal, and it's much more responsibly harvested than the imported stuff.

When you shop for king crab, whatever the label says, ask whether it comes from Alaska or if it's imported. Approximately 70% of the king crab sold in the U.S. is imported, so it's important to make that distinction and go domestic.

Shark Why It's Bad: Problems associated with our eating too many sharks happen at all stages of the food chain,. For one, these predatory fish are extremely high in mercury, which poses threats to humans. But ocean ecosystems suffer, too. "With fewer sharks around, the species they eat, like cownose rays and jellyfish, have increased in numbers,". "And the rays are eating—and depleting—scallops and other fish." There are fewer of those fish in the oceans for us to eat, placing an economic strain on coastal communities that depend on those fisheries.

Among the recommendations for shark alternatives are Pacific halibut and Atlantic mackerel.

Orange Roughy Why It's Bad: In addition to having high levels of mercury, orange roughy can take between 20 and 40 years to reach full maturity and reproduces late in life, which makes it difficult for populations to recover from overfishing. Orange roughy has such a reputation for being overharvested that some large restaurant chains, including Red Lobster, refuse to serve it. However, it still pops up in grocer freezers, sometimes mislabeled as "sustainably harvested." There are no fisheries of orange roughy that are considered well-managed or are certified by the Marine Stewardship Council, so avoid any that you see.

Opt, for yellow snapper or domestic catfish to get the same texture as orange roughy in your recipes.

Atlantic Bluefin Tuna Why It's Bad: A recent analysis by *The New York Times* found that Atlantic bluefin tuna has the highest levels of mercury of any type of tuna. To top it off, bluefin tuna are severely overharvested, to the point of reaching near-extinction levels, and are considered "critically endangered" by the International Union for Conservation of Nature. Rather than trying to navigate the ever-changing recommendations for which tuna is best, consider giving it up altogether and switching to a healthy, flavorful alternative, such as Alaska wild-caught salmon.

If you really can't give up tuna, opt for American or Canadian (but not imported!) albacore tuna, which is caught while it's young and doesn't contain as high levels of mercury.

Chilean Sea Bass Why It's Bad: Most Chilean sea bass sold in the US comes from fishermen who have captured them illegally, although the US Department of State says that illegal harvesting of the fish has declined in recent years. Nevertheless, fish stocks are in such bad shape that the nonprofit Greenpeace estimates that, unless people stop eating this fish, the entire species could be commercially extinct within five years. Food and Water Watch's guide notes that these fish are high in mercury, as well.

These fish are very popular and considered a delicacy, but you can get the same texture and feel with US hook-and-line-caught haddock.

Why Women Shouldn't Eat Factory-Farmed Chicken

More than just a food-safety threat, contaminated chicken has been pegged as the culprit in a common uncomfortable condition.

Tests from the nonprofit Consumers Union have found that grocery store shelves are littered with contaminated meat. Their tests regularly show that as much as two-thirds of grocery-store chicken contains bacteria resistant to some of the most common classes of antibiotics.

While those tests have an obvious ick factor, they also prove that dirty factory farms are filling our guts with bacteria that can cause all sorts of infections. And for women, that could mean more uncomfortable urinary tract infections (UTIs).

In 80 to 90 percent of routine urinary tract infections, *E. coli* is the most common cause.

Supermarket chicken could be where all that *E. coli* is coming from.

People are eating a lot more chicken because it's often perceived as healthier, But what people don't realize is that chicken is pretty heavily contaminated with bacteria in general, and those bacteria tend to be drug resistant.

The authors collected urine samples from women in Canada and California who had been diagnosed with UTIs and compared the *E. coli* bacteria in those samples with *E. coli* found in samples of beef, pork, and chicken purchased at grocery stores in those same regions. They also collected *E. coli* samples from animals killed at commercial slaughterhouses.

In 71 percent of the cases, the *E. coli* bacteria collected from women with UTIs matched that of the *E. coli* found in the supermarket chicken, while just 29 percent matched those found in beef and pork. Similarly, the *E. coli* bacteria collected from factory-farm slaughterhouse chickens matched UTI bacteria 79 percent of the time, compared to just 3 percent of those from cattle and 17 percent of those from pigs.

When you eat the meat, these bacteria live in your gut, that bacteria can cause a UTI as much as six months after you've eaten contaminated chicken.

In the second half of the study, they analyzed the strains of *E. coli* found in women suffering UTIs and the supermarket chicken for its resistance to the antibiotics commonly used to treat UTIs, and she found that some of the bacteria had developed, or were developing, resistance to the medications.

"Drug-resistant UTIs are more difficult to treat," "Most of what they found could be treated with antibiotics, but it's still concerning because that just means we have fewer drugs to treat them."

The researchers are joining the chorus of food activists and physicians who would like the Food and Drug Administration (FDA) to tighten restrictions on the levels and types of antibiotics that feedlot operators are permitted to add to feed and inject into animals. "Anytime you use antibiotics, we're just more concerned with these *E. coli* ending up in people at some point.

The FDA took baby steps towards antibiotic overuse in January, when they restricted the use of antibiotics in animals raised for food. Those same antibiotics are one of four types commonly used to treat UTIs. But that announcement came weeks after the FDA withdrew a petition that would have allowed it to regulate the use of the two most commonly used antibiotics, penicillin and tetracycline. So the risk of antibiotic resistance is still dire.

The bottom line? If you're prone to UTIs, buy organic chicken. Research published in the journal *Environmental Health Perspectives* found that turkeys and chickens raised on organic poultry farms had almost four times lower levels of drug-resistant bacteria in their systems than those raised on cramped, dirty feedlots.

Better still, get your organic chicken from a local farmer. On both organic and feedlot farms, the amount of bacteria, studies have found, is directly related to the size of the flock. Local farmers with small flocks of chickens that roam on pasture and eat a healthy diet of bugs, grass, and organic grain will have the lowest levels of bacteria, drug resistant or otherwise.

There's Arsenic in Your Chicken

Nearly four years — yes, *four years* — after the Center for Food Safety filed a petition with the FDA calling for the withdrawal of arsenic-laced feed given to chickens, turkeys, and pigs, the FDA has finally responded. Actually, it responded to the lawsuit that the CFS subsequently filed, demanding that the agency respond to the citizen petition.

Better late than never, right? But the response was bittersweet. The FDA only agreed to withdraw three of the four arsenicals on the market

The fourth drug, nitarsone, is still allowed in the feed supply. As for what makes nitarsone "safer" than the other arsenicals being banned, that part is still unclear.

Arsenic-containing compounds were first approved for commercial use in medicated animal feed in the 1940s. Their purpose was to promote faster growth in poultry and increased feed efficiency ... essentially, fatter chickens that don't eat as much. If animal feed produced by the pharmaceutical industry doesn't already make you shudder, ponder this: A 2006 report by the Institute for Agriculture and Trade Policy found that over 70% of the 8.7 billion American broiler chickens produced each year have been fed arsenic, and some of that arsenic stays in the chicken meat.

The poultry industry has claimed that the arsenic fed to their birds has no adverse health effects on the consumer. This is because the kind of arsenic used in feed additives is "organic" arsenic, which is arguably less toxic than "inorganic" arsenic, a known carcinogen. But even the FDA acknowledges that recent studies have found that organic arsenic has the ability to convert to inorganic arsenic in animal tissue — the animal tissue that you eat.

While poultry companies claim the amount of arsenic detected in chicken meat is too low to be of any concern, consider that the easier availability and lower cost of modern poultry production means the average American now eats a lot more chicken than ever before. From 1965 to 2013, consumption of chicken jumped from 33.7 pounds to 83.1 pounds per person per year: a 250% increase. And that raises the question: Just how much arsenic in our systems is *too* much? And what effect does it have on children versus adults?

The FDA claims it is continuing to evaluate nitarsone, the last remaining arsenical making its rounds in the poultry industry, and will make a final decision on whether or not to pull it from the food supply in 2014.

Diabetic neuropathy now affects an estimated 15-18 million Americans. That means that close to 70% of the almost 26 million Americans with type 2 diabetes suffer from this sometimes-debilitating condition. And while there are approximately 100 different causes of neuropathy, diabetes ranks highest on the list, accounting for a full one third of neuropathy cases.

Symptoms associated with diabetic neuropathy can be quite aggressive and include pain, loss of sensation, tingling and even weakness, typically affecting hands and feet.

Clinicians and researchers in Europe have long known about the effectiveness of a common nutritional supplement, alpha-lipoic acid, as an effective approach to diabetic neuropathy. But here in America most patients are given pharmaceuticals to treat the symptoms. And yet, wonderful clinical data now confirms the profound effectiveness of alpha-lipoic acid in treating diabetic neuropathy.

Both the well-conducted research as well as my own clinical experience in using this nonprescription approach to treating diabetic neuropathy will keep alpha-lipoic acid in my tool kit.

Lipoic acid is a potent and protective antioxidant that is both fat and water-soluble. That means it can penetrate virtually all of the body's tissues, including the brain and nerves. In addition, it acts as a heavy metal chelator, helping the body rid itself of toxic metals like lead and mercury. It also helps maintain levels of another brain important antioxidant, *glutathione.*

7 Facts You Didn't Know About Calcium

I'm thrilled to share with you seven facts about calcium that you may not know, and that could make a big difference in the way you benefit from this crucial supplement.

So, let's get started!

1. The name "calcium" is derived from Latin.

Calx or calcis is Latin for "lime." This makes sense since calcium is extracted from limestone, and also from marble and chalk. Of the elements that make up the earth's crust, calcium is the fifth most abundant one.

In nature, calcium is never found in its pure form; its molecular structure causes it to attach itself to other elements to form compounds. This is why you usually see calcium referred to with another element in the name: calcium carbonate, calcium citrate, calcium sulfate, and so forth. Because of this binding characteristic, calcium is used in industry to remove oxygen, sulfur, and carbon from alloys.

2. Diets high in animal protein and phosphorous-rich foods like soft drinks and cow's milk inhibit calcium absorption.

Animal protein is acidifying, and the body therefore uses calcium to neutralize the acidic environment caused by its consumption, especially when bicarbonate reserves are depleted. So, in essence, the calcium that is used to neutralize the acid never makes it into your bones.

Phosphorus, which is found in acidifying foods and beverages like soft drinks (phosphoric acid) and cow's milk, also has a detrimental effect. The debilitating effects of phosphorous on bone are well-documented – the jaw disease known as osteonecrosis of the jaw (ONJ) was once called "phossy jaw" because of its clear correlation with phosphorous exposure. And of course, the most widely-prescribed osteoporosis drugs are phosphorous-based bisphosphonates, which artificially alter bone metabolism, making it brittle and prone to fracture.

3. Calcium from vegetables is better absorbed than calcium in cow's milk.

A recent study compared the absorption rate of calcium from kale and from milk, and the results were clear: the calcium from kale was absorbed at a rate of 40.9%, whereas the calcium from milk was absorbed at a rate of 32.1%. Kale is an especially good plant source for calcium absorption because of its low oxalate content.

4. You lose calcium from your bones as you sleep.

Interestingly, calcium loss occurs at a higher rate during the night, with women losing more as they sleep than men. According to a study published in the Journal of Clinical Endocrinology and Metabolism, this may be due to a difference between the sexes' parathyroid (PTH) levels at night. PTH monitors blood calcium levels, and men tend to increase their PTH production at night, whereas women do not.

5. Smaller doses of calcium are best.

While the Medical Establishment tends to prescribe massive doses of calcium as a treatment for osteoporosis (and they often prescribe the wrong kind of calcium – more on that later), your body is actually unable to absorb more than 500mg of calcium at a time. However, you need more than 500mg per day, so that's why I recommend spreading your calcium intake throughout the day.

6. Calcium helps far more than just your bones.

It's also necessary for the proper functioning of muscles and nerves, and amazingly, calcium facilitates communication between the brain and every part of your body. Calcium also plays a role in your circulatory system by mediating the expansion and constriction of blood vessels (vasodilation and vasoconstriction).

And here's another important function of calcium: it helps with the release of insulin and stabilizes and optimizes various enzymes.

In short, calcium affects the functioning of your entire body.

7. Overconsumption of calcium carbonate or any form of inorganic calcium can cause major health problems and unpleasant side effects.

The irony is, calcium carbonate is the form usually prescribed by doctors; but it's one of the least absorbable forms of this mineral, and therein lies the problem. Another commonly prescribed form of inorganic calcium is calcium citrate.

When calcium carbonate is ingested, very little is absorbed into your bones, especially if other synergistic minerals and vitamins (such as magnesium and Vitamin D) are not consumed in proportion to the calcium. That's why large amounts taken in isolation are particularly dangerous – it simply increases the amount of unabsorbed calcium in your body. This excess calcium then gets deposited in soft tissues, contributing to the formation of kidney stones, artery blockage, and the development of hypercalcemia.

Additionally, consuming excessive inorganic calcium can cause side effects such as nausea, gastrointestinal discomfort, constipation, fatigue, and a general feeling of weakness.

The vast majority of kidney stones are comprised mostly of calcium oxalate, leading researchers to believe that calcium supplements contribute to kidney stones. However, as I mentioned above, calcium from food sources does not cause kidney stones. That's because the calcium in foods is organic, and therefore bioavailable.

So, Should I Take Calcium Supplements Or Not?

While food sources are ideal, it's nearly impossible to get all the calcium you need from food alone, especially if you want to build your bones. It comes down to finding the right calcium supplement – one that's bioavailable, organic, plant-based, and doesn't come in a high dosage. Calcium Microcrystalline Hydroxyapatite is an excellent source and very bioavailable.

What Your Nails Say About Your Health?

Thinking of those ugly white spots, unsightly ridges and sometimes crumbling and splitting nails, do you think that your nails could be telling you something about your state of physical health and general well-being? Almost like the eyes being the window to the soul?

Historically speaking, women who were from the high class grew their nails as this showed to the world that servants did their work and that they were proper ladies. Today it is not a case of class anymore, but a telltale sign of meticulous grooming, and a greatly featuring fashion accessory. Nail décor has almost become a subsection of the arts. The fact that nails have a true and real function has almost been forgotten.

Nails are part of the skin, which in its totality is a complex and vital organ. The visible part of the nail is made up of several layers of dead compacted keratin (the same substance that hooves and horns are made of). This fibrous protein turns into a tough, flexible shield, acting as protection to the fingertip and underlying soft tissue, and is an excellent tool for small scraping and scratching jobs. The thin strip of skin running along the nail bed or otherwise known as the cuticle, in its turn grants protection to the living keratin cells responsible for the continuous growth of the nail. Often this skin is pushed back in the name of beauty, but more harm than good is done. Bad habits like biting the nails or ripping off the bits of skin, can damage the nail bed, creating a perfect gateway and fertile breeding ground for viruses and bacteria. It is often thought that the nail is an impermeable barrier, but surprisingly, it is very sensitive to water and chemicals which can easily ruin healthy nails as can be often seen on the hands of hairdressers. While keeping all these obvious causes in mind, one should never forget that spots, ridges, discolored and splitting nails could very well be a way of one's body urging you to do some inspection.

With emphasis on "could be", the color of one's nails could be (but is not necessarily) an indication of a medical problem. A healthy nail has a rosy shine to it. Another sign of a healthy nail is a smooth surface.

Signals Our Nails Are Sending

Pale or white nails could mean anemia, kidney failure, heart failure or malnourishment but normally there are far more prominent symptoms that lead the way to such a serious diagnosis.

White nails with yellow edges along the nail bed could be a symptom of a liver abnormality or hepatitis.

Blue or purple nails could be a symptom of oxygen deprivation as in the case of pneumonia, asthma or emphysema or it could simply be a sign of being cold.

A **vaguely blueish tint** could indicate diabetes, but once again, it could also have no cause.

Yellow nails (usually with ridges) often indicate a fungal infection but could also be the result of frequent use of acetone to remove nail polish, glue for false nails or other harsh chemicals.

White spots are mostly caused by minor injuries on the nail bed and appear without one even knowing where and when, which will disappear with a bit of patience, as it will eventually grow out. Sometimes though, deficiencies can cause these spots. Vitamin C, zinc and calcium are common culprits, but also a protein deficiency may be responsible.

Horizontal ridges could be an early manifestation of psoriasis or arthritis, but in both cases, it is usually accompanied by a red-brownish discoloration of the nail itself. It could also be a harmless temporary or permanent condition caused by trauma to the nail bed for example accidentally bringing down the hammer on the fingernail rather than on the head of the "nail".

Should one's **nails break, split or crumble easily** if you are not constantly exposing your hands to water or chemicals, then it could be that your thyroid gland is playing up, but there are many other more significant symptoms such as hair loss, that would probably emerge long before the nails become an issue.

Don't forget that the shape of the nail may be of some importance. When nails turn upwards and form a **spoon-like shape**, which is sometimes enough to hold a few drops of water, the person has "spoon nails" or koilonychia as the condition is known in the medical world. This can be linked to a variety of diseases including heart disease and cancer, but on the other hand can be hereditary and completely innocent.

Generally speaking the nails can give some sort of indication of one's health, but mostly deviations from what is seen as a healthy nail mean absolutely nothing. If you should happen to have any reason for concern, see your doctor, but remember that white nails don't automatically mean that you have heart failure, and splitting nails is no definite for a hypoactive thyroid gland. In the meantime, it is a great idea to treat your nails with respect, trim them gently, clean and moisturize them regularly and enjoy them pure and simple, pink and smooth.

CoQ10 & Grass-fed Meat

COQ10 is an essential nutrient both synthesized by the body and taken from diet. Studies show that our bodies typically produce plenty until we turn 20 thereafter, production diminishes, and many adults over 40 show deficiencies.

CoQ10 deficiencies are associated with atherosclerosis (hardening of arteries), heart disease, diabetes and high blood pressure. Many people have supplemented with CoQ10 to treat ailments including heart failure, high blood pressure, Parkinson's disease and diabetes.

The enzyme plays a vital role in metabolism and production of energy. It also may be crucial for brain function, cognition and memory. It's a powerful antioxidant, preventing DNA damage and helping to prevent LDL oxidation, which is now considered a key marker for heart disease.

The richest sources of **CoQ10** are red meats, especially the organ meats. Because the body makes less with age, we need to replenish through diet. But grain-fed cattle may produce meat with up to **10 times less CoQ10** than those grass-fed.

Unless you regularly consume wild game or eat internal organs of grass-fed animals...it is difficult to maintain good blood levels of CoQ10 from dietary sources alone.

Daily Dose?

Recommended dosage is typically from 30 to 90mg daily, but some are recommended treatments as high as 200mg/day.

Benefits of Grass-Fed Beef

When compared to the steroid and antibiotic pumped grain-fed beef, organic grass-fed beef:

- Provides up to four times Omega-3 fats
- Is lower in overall fat and calories, some by as much as 100 calories less per serving
- Is up to 5 times more concentrated with conjugated linoleic acid (contributes to heart health, decreases cancer risk, helps to burn fat, and used to prevent and treat diabetes)
- Has shown far less (some say "zero") risk of carrying Mad Cow disease

If you don't have access or prefer not to eat grass-fed red meats, or wild game such as elk or deer, heart health pros recommend taking a CoQ10 supplement along with a healthy oil, such as fish oil (for better absorption). If you are on statin drugs, experts say you **absolutely** should be supplementing with CoQ10.

7 Facts About Roundup

1. **You're eating it—in "excessive" levels.** The majority of glyphosate dumped onto American land each year isn't in yards—it's on your food crops. The most popular genetically engineered (GE) crops planted on millions of U.S. acres each year are designed to withstand heavy dousing of glyphosate. Chemical companies are making a killing on this, since they produce both the unnatural GE seed *and* the chemical that needs to be used on those seeds. But glyphosate is a systemic chemical, meaning it's taken up inside of the plants that we—and farm animals—eat. This spring, Norwegian scientists studying U.S. soy found "excessive" levels of glyphosate *inside* of the food crop. Don't eat tofu? Doesn't matter: GE corn and soy fall under dozens of different ingredient names in most processed foods.
2. **It doubles your risk of lymphoma.** A major new review of 44 scientific studies found that glyphosate exposure doubles farmers' risk of developing non-Hodgkin's lymphoma. The study authors theorize that glyphosate disrupts the normal functioning of white blood cells, throwing your immune system into a sickened, dysfunctional state.
3. **It's raining Roundup.** Each year, nonorganic farmers dump millions of pounds of glyphosate on food crops. The levels are so excessive, that the federal scientists recently detected the weed killer in the air and rain. Veteran pesticide-exposure scientist Warren

Porter, PhD, professor of environmental toxicology and zoology at the University of Wisconsin–Madison, crunched the numbers and found the data collected by the United States Geological Survey scientists reveal exposure that could potentially alter your hormones, leading to obesity, heart problems, and diabetes.

4. **It's annihilating monarchs.** Researchers at Iowa State University found that the heavy use of glyphosate has resulted in an 81 percent decrease in the monarch butterfly population. Traditionally, milkweed—the plants monarchs need to reproduce and survive as a species—would rebound after farmers used cultivation to kill weeds, but chemical interventions wipe the plant out. Organic agriculture bans the use of chemical pesticides, so every dollar you shift to organic helps save their foodstuff and more monarch butterflies.
5. **It flat-out kills human cells.** In 2009, French researchers published a scientific paper in the journal *Chemical Research in Toxicology* showing that low levels of four glyphosate formulations used in Roundup—levels far below what's allowed in agriculture; levels on par with what's in our food—all kill human umbilical, embryonic, and placental cells within 24 hours.
6. **It's killing your gut.** Glyphosate isn't just an herbicide; it's registered as an antimicrobial agent in the U.S., too, thanks to its ability to wipe out a wide variety of pathogenic organisms. The problem is harmful pathogens like *Clostridium botulinum*, Salmonella, and E. coli are able to survive glyphosate in the gut, but the "good guys" in your digestive tract, protective microorganisms, bacillus and lactobacillus, for instance, are killed off. This *could* set your digestive tract up for a nightmarish situation, including "leaky gut," where the protective gut lining is compromised, allowing bacteria and toxins to escape into your bloodstream.
7. **It doesn't work.** The kicker? *It's not working!* Genetically engineering crop seeds to live through herbicide sprayings that would normally kill the crop is a failed technology and a losing battle. Just as overusing antibiotics led to hard-to-kill, antibiotic-resistant supergerms, abusing weed killers has fueled the emergence of nearly impossible-to-kill superweeds.

When GE technology was first introduced, chemical companies touted it as a way to *reduce* chemical use on food crops. But Professor Chuck Benbrook, PhD, a research professor at Washington State University, recently found that between 1996 and 2011, GMO technology actually *increased* herbicide use by 527 million pounds—that's an 11 percent bump. And for every pound less of insecticide used, farmers used four pounds more of herbicides.

Because glyphosate-resistant GE crops are failing miserably, the Environmental Protection Agency (EPA)—right now—is considering the approval of an even nastier GE seed designed to survive dousing of glyphosate *and* the highly toxic, older 2,4-D weed killer. This is called "stacking," and it's expected to dramatically increase the amount of 2,4-D used on our food. In fact, approving crops genetically engineered to survive repeated dousing of 2,4-D will likely *quadruple* pesticide use, according to Dave Mortensen, PhD, weed scientist at Penn State University. That's bad news, considering 2,4-D has been linked to hypothyroidism, suppressed immune function, Parkinson's disease, and cancer, among other ills.

So how can we get Roundup out of the air, soil, and our bodies? There's only one way: **buy organic food**. In doing so, you're sending farmers a clear message.

The Best Foods for Your Liver

Foods for your liver are essential to keeping your body's powerhouse—your liver—functioning optimally. A healthy liver plays a key role in relieving digestive issues, such as a sluggish metabolism, gas, bloating, and constipation. It regulates blood sugar levels, which—when out of balance—can cause sugar cravings, fatigue, and fuzzy thinking.

A toxic liver can lead to inflammatory diseases, such as diabetes, arthritis, high blood pressure, and autoimmune diseases. Without a healthy liver, you may suffer from hormonal imbalances that can cause headaches, mood swings, and depression. It's time to nurture this amazing organ!

Use these foods for your liver to start feeling better:

Water After oxygen, your body needs water more than any other substance, including food, just to survive. Because water flushes toxins and waste products from your body, you feel more energized and alert when your body is fully hydrated (which most of us usually aren't!). Usually eight to 10, 8-ounce glasses will do the trick. Skip the ice when you're drinking water in between meals. Your body uses energy to warm the ice, diluting important digestive enzymes.

Crucifers Crucifers contain vital phytonutrients——to help your liver neutralize chemicals, pesticides, drugs, and carcinogens. Crucifer foods include broccoli, cabbage, cauliflower, bok choy, and daikon, a root rich in phenolic compounds that could prevent the formation of carcinogen in your stomach in response to foods made with hydrogenated oils and sodium nitrite.

Dark Leafy Greens Kale, Brussels sprouts, and cabbage are powerful brassica vegetables that contain high levels of sulfur, which supports your liver in its detoxification process, triggering it to remove free radicals and other toxic chemicals.

Dandelion is another dark leafy green known as one of the most effective and recommended plants to support liver detoxification. One of its chemical components, taraxacin, is believed to stimulate the digestive organs and trigger the liver and gallbladder to release bile, which supports digestion and fat absorption.

Sea Vegetables One of the oldest inhabitants of the earth, sea vegetables detoxify your body by preventing assimilation of heavy metals, such as cadmium, as well as other environmental toxins. Studies at McGill University have revealed that a compound in brown algae reduced the uptake of radioactive particles into bone.

Sprouted Seeds, Nuts, Beans, and Grains The energy contained in a seed, grain, nut, or legume is ignited through soaking and sprouting. And those sprouts are superhigh in enzymes, proteins that act as catalysts for all of your body's functions. Broccoli sprouts appear to be in sulforaphane, which triggers your body's natural cancer protection.

Sulfur-Rich Foods *Garlic*—One of the oldest land-based medicinal foods on the planet, garlic contains an active sulfur-based compound called allicin, a critical supporter of liver detoxification. It helps your liver rid your body of mercury, certain food additives, and the hormone estrogen.

Onions, shallots, and leeks—A relative of garlic, these foods also contain those smelly sulfur compounds that support your liver in its production of glutathione, the compound in every cell of your body that neutralizes free radicals.

Eggs—Eggs provide some of the highest-quality protein, containing all eight essential amino acids, cholesterol, and the essential nutrient choline. Your liver needs these essential amino acids to perform detoxification processes. Choline a coenzyme needed for metabolism, is found in the egg yolk and protects your liver from a wide range of toxic substances, while detoxifying heavy metals.

Artichokes—Two phytonutrients found in artichokes, cynarin and silymarin, have been shown to nourish your liver, increase bile production, and prevent gallstones.

Mushrooms—Maitake, shiitake, and reishi mushrooms are thought to provide significant healing nutrients that nourish and support your immune system. These mushrooms contain a powerful antioxidant which neutralizes free radicals while increasing enzymes that boost antioxidant activity.

Fruits *Berries*—Blueberries, strawberries, raspberries, and cranberries are among nature's superfoods because they contain phytochemicals—antioxidant-rich plant compounds that help your liver protect your body from free radicals and oxidative stress, which have been linked to chronic diseases and aging. Anthocyanin and polyphenols found in berries have been shown to inhibit the proliferation of cancer cells in the liver.

Apples—Apples, like berries, contain powerful phenolic compounds, including flavonoids, which can fight inflammatory disease. They also contain pectin, a valuable source of soluble fiber than can help eliminate toxic buildup.

Prebiotic-Rich Foods

Prebiotics are indigestible fibers that feed your beneficial gut flora, known as probiotics. Probiotics are living microorganisms that support your health and wellbeing. Prebiotics are nonliving dietary fibers that help probiotics grow and flourish. Prebiotics are found in asparagus, leeks, cruciferous vegetables, and several root vegetables—burdock, chicory, dandelion, beets, and Jerusalem artichoke.

Cultured Foods

These include kimchi—a traditional Korean dish made of fermented cabbage, radish, garlic, red pepper, onion, ginger, and salt—and sauerkraut. Fermentation, an ancient form of preservation in which food is naturally transformed by microorganisms that break down all the food's carbohydrates and protein, aids in digestion, thanks to a plethora of healthy bacteria like lactobacilli. Real miso_is another example of fermented food.

Healthy Fats

Flax seeds—A great source of eomega-3 essential fatty acids, these seeds help regulate hormone levels.

Hemp seeds—A mix of clean omega-6 and omega-3 fats, these seeds help ease inflammation while lowering dangerous blood fat levels.

Chia seeds—A staple in Central American Aztec and Mayan diets for thousands of years, these seeds are all-around nutritional powerhouses. Three tablespoons contain 5 grams of protein, 200 milligrams of calcium, 10 grams of healthy fat, and 12 grams of fiber.

Coconut oil—An extremely healthy saturated fat, coconut oil is easy to digest and is almost immediately broken down by enzymes in your saliva and gastric juices. This means pancreatic fat-digesting enzymes are not essential, which produces less strain on your liver so it can work more efficiently.

Avocado—A vital source of monounsaturated fat rich in oleic acid, avocados contain glutathione, an essential nutrient for liver health.

Cold-pressed, unrefined extra-virgin olive oil—Unadulterated olive oil is rich in phenols, the same anti-inflammatory compounds found in berries and apples. Daily consumption of olive oil supports the liver in decreasing oxidative stress in the body.

Herbs

Ginger—Gingerol antioxidants possess anti-inflammatory, antiviral, and antimicrobial properties. Ginger supports detoxification by nourishing your liver, promoting circulation, unclogging blocked arteries, and lowering blood cholesterol by as much as 30 percent.

Cumin—In one Indian study, cumin was shown to boost the liver's detoxification power while stimulating the secretion of enzymes from the pancreas, which helps your system absorb nutrients.

Coriander—Coriander seeds have been shown to help the liver lower blood lipids among those with obesity and diabetes, lowering triglycerides and LDL (bad) cholesterol, while increasing HDL (good) cholesterol.

Fresh cilantro leaves help remove heavy metals from the body, mobilizing mercury, cadmium, lead, and aluminum that's been stored in the brain, spinal cord, and central nervous system so your body can eliminate them.

Cardamom—This member of the ginger family helps improve digestion by stimulating the flow of bile, which is critical in fat metabolism. It accelerates the gastric emptying rate, relaxing the stomach valves that prevent food from entering the small intestine, allowing nutrients to pass on to the small intestine without excess effort.

Cayenne—This detoxer stimulates your circulatory system, increasing the pulse of your lymphatic and digestive rhythms, heating your body. This "heat" helps get your gastric juices flowing, enhancing your body's ability to metabolize food and toxins.

Cinnamon—Used for centuries for flavoring and medicine, cinnamon keeps sticky platelets from forming clots in your arteries, boosts metabolism, and prevents candida, a condition characterized by yeast overgrowth.

Fennel—The essential oils in fennel prompt the secretion of gastric juices, helping to lower inflammation in your digestive tract and diminish aide product. This allows your body to absorb nutrients more efficiently.

Turmeric—The curcumin compounds in turmeric have been shown to heal your liver, aiding in detoxification and strengthening your whole body.

Animal Protein

Experiment to see what protein sources make you feel energized, satisfied, and balanced. For most of our existence, we've depended on nutrient-rich dietary fats in the form of meats, fatty fish, and bone marrow for at least 60 percent of our caloric consumption. Factory farms and industrialized ingredients changed all that, and in 1912, heart disease the medical community identified heart disease.

Meat—Eat only clean, grass-fed land animals, ones raised without the use of feed grown with pesticides. Avoid factory-farmed meat laden with chemicals, hormones, and antibiotics.

Fish—In general, fish is healthy and protein-rich. Some wild-caught fish, such as Atlantic mackerel from Canada, sardines, and anchovies, are notable for their omega-3 fatty acids and their low level of contaminants. Wild salmon, an excellent source of protein, is also one of the best sources of omega-3 fatty acids from the krill and shrimp they eat—that's what gives salmon their beautiful color and makes them rich in antioxidants.

Vegetable Protein We need to eat protein to build new cells, maintain tissue, and synthesize new proteins to perform basic bodily functions. You *can* do it with vegetarian sources of protein.

Marine-based—Microalgae contains protein, along with high levels of chlorophyll, which helps heal you by removing toxic drug deposits and heavy metals in your body, improve liver function, and neutralize carcinogens.

Land-based—Cooked lentils, chickpeas, and black, kidney, and pinto beans contain about 15 grams of protein per cup. A quarter cup of sunflower seeds pack 6 grams of protein. Greens count, too. Eating a cup each of cooked spinach and broccoli equals about 9 grams of protein.

Top Tips to Decrease Your Breast Cancer Risk

Breast cancer is probably one of the most feared diagnosis a woman can get. The mere mention of it conjures up images of death, despair, or at best, disfigurement.

According to breastcancer.org,1 one in eight women will develop invasive breast cancer in her lifetime, and nearly 40,000 women lose their lives to the disease each year.

With such odds stacked against you, what, if anything, can you do to prevent becoming a statistic? In truth, there are many measures you can take—each of which will help decrease your risk.

It's important to realize that less than 10 percent of all breast cancer cases are thought to be related to genetic risk factors. The remainder—90 percent—appear to be triggered by environmental factors.

I strongly believe that cancer is preventable through appropriate lifestyle changes, such as cleaning up your diet, optimizing your vitamin D levels, exercising, and avoiding toxins from every source you can.

This means taking careful inventory of the household and personal care products you use, and the furnishings and other potentially toxic items you get into contact with on a daily basis. Toxic overexposure undoubtedly play a *major* role in cancer development, and recent studies are finally starting to shed light on the worst offenders.

Scientists Identify 'Highest Priority' Toxins for Breast Cancer Prevention

According to recent research published in the National Institutes of Health (NIH) journal, *Environmental Health Perspectives,* you can reduce your risk of breast cancer by avoiding certain chemicals found in common, everyday products.

"Because the study found that animal tests are able to predict likely human breast carcinogens, the new report could serve as a major step forward in breast cancer prevention, expanding the list of possible breast cancer triggers. That's especially important because only about 10 percent of breast cancers are genetic in nature—scientists believe environment plays a huge role...

'Every woman in America has been exposed to chemicals that may increase her risk of getting breast cancer. Unfortunately, the link between toxic chemicals and breast cancer has largely been ignored,' says Julia Brody, PhD, study author and executive director at Silent Spring Institute. 'Reducing chemical exposures could save many, many women's lives.'"

In a previous study, the researchers had identified 216 chemicals that increase mammary gland tumors in rodents. In this paper, they narrowed the focus to 102 chemicals that large numbers of women are exposed to on a regular basis, through food, medications, air pollution, or consumer products.

They then prioritized the chemicals, and grouped them based on exposure, carcinogenic potential, and chemical structure. This sorting resulted in 17 chemical groups of related chemicals, which were flagged as "high priority" due to their ability to consistently produce mammary tumors in animal tests.

Top Offenders

Their list of cancer-causing chemical groups to avoid, and their most common sources of exposure, includes the following. Another 27 different carcinogens that do not fit into the chemical categories listed below are also considered high priority. These chemicals include certain ones found in pesticides, consumer products, and food.

Two examples of the latter are methyl eugenol, which is used in processed food as a natural and artificial flavoring, and nitrosamines in smoked meats. The researchers also list obesity and medical radiation as preventable risk factors, the latter of which would include unnecessary mammograms.

High Priority Chemicals to Avoid for Breast Cancer Prevention

Flame retardants: Flame retardant products, polyester resins, plastic polymers, and rigid polyurethane foams	**Acrylamide:** Diet (especially starchy foods, such as French fries, cooked at high temperatures), tobacco smoke, and polyacrylamide gels in consumer products, such as diapers
Aromatic amines: Polyurethane, pesticides, Azo dyes, and many other products	**Benzene:** Gasoline (riding in a car, pumping gasoline, and storing gasoline in a basement or attached garage), tobacco smoke, adhesive removers, paints, sealants, finishers, and engine fuel and oils
Halogenated organic solvents: Dry cleaning, hair spray propellant, soil fumigants, food processing, gasoline additives, and paint and spot removers	**Ethylene (EtO) and propylene oxide (PO):** EtO is a gas used to sterilize medical equipment, food and spices, clothing, and musical instruments. Also found in tobacco smoke and auto exhaust. PO is a sterilant and fumigant. Also found in automotive and paint products

1,3-Butadiene: Cigarette smoke, automobile exhaust, gasoline fumes, and emissions from industrial facilities	**Heterocyclic amines:** Meat cooked at high temperatures, and tobacco smoke
Endogenous and pharmaceutical hormones and other endocrine disrupting chemicals: Estrogens, progesterone, and DES, along with other hormones	**Non-hormonal pharmaceuticals that have hormonal activity:** These include four chemotherapeutic agents, two veterinary drugs possibly present in food, the diuretic furosemide, the anti-fungal griseofulvin, and several anti-infective agents
MX: One of hundreds of genotoxic by-products of drinking water disinfection	**Perfluorooctanoic acid PFOA:** Non-stick and stain-resistant coatings on rugs, furniture, clothes and cookware; fire-fighting applications, cosmetics, lubricants, paints, and adhesives
Nitro-PAHs: Air pollution, primarily from diesel exhaust	**PAHs:** Tobacco smoke, air pollution, and charred foods
Ochratoxin A (a naturally occurring mycotoxin): Contaminated grain, nuts, and pork products	**Styrene:** Food that has been in contact with polystyrene; consumer products and building materials, including polystyrene, carpets, adhesives, hobby and craft supplies, and home maintenance products

Flame Retardants Do FAR More Harm Than Good...

While it's difficult to single out any particular chemical grouping as being "the worst," fire retardants may fit the bill by the fact that they are used in so many furnishings, including your mattress, where you spend a significant portion of your life. *"The average American baby is born with 10 fingers, 10 toes and the highest recorded levels of flame retardants among infants in the world. The toxic chemicals are present in nearly every home, packed into couches, chairs and many other products. Two powerful industries — Big Tobacco and chemical manufacturers — waged deceptive campaigns that led to the proliferation of these chemicals, which don't even work as promised."*

An estimated 90 percent of Americans have flame-retardant chemicals in their bodies, and *many* studies have linked them to human health risks, including infertility, birth defects, lower IQ scores, behavioral problems in children, as well as liver, kidney, testicular, and breast cancers.

Flame-retardant chemicals belong to the same class of chemicals as DDT and PCBs (organohalogens), and like the former, they, too, build up in the environment. These chemicals also react with other toxins as they burn to produce cancer-causing dioxins. The chemical industry claims that fire-retardant furniture increases escape time in a fire by 15-fold.

In reality, this claim came from a study using powerful, NASA-style flame retardants, which provided an extra 15 seconds of escape time. But this is not the same type of chemical used in most furniture, and government and independent studies show that the most widely used flame-retardant chemicals provide no benefit for people while *increasing* the amounts of toxic chemicals in smoke.

A flame-retardant chemical known as chlorinated tris (TDCPP) was *removed* from children's pajamas in the 1970s amid concerns that it may cause cancer, but now it's a ubiquitous addition to couch cushions across the United States. As for your mattress, I recommend getting one that's either made of 100% wool or Kevlar, both of which are natural flame retardant without added chemicals.

Antiperspirants and Cosmetics—Other Major Culprits

Parabens are chemicals that serve as preservatives in antiperspirants and many cosmetics, as well as sun lotions. Previous studies have shown that all parabens have estrogenic activity in human breast cancer cells. Research published in 20126 found one or more paraben esters in 99 percent of the 160 tissue samples collected from 40 mastectomies. The consistent presence of parabens in cancerous human breast tissue suggests antiperspirants and other cosmetics may also increase your risk of breast cancer.

While antiperspirants are a common source of parabens, the authors note that the source of the parabens cannot be established, and that seven of the 40 patients reportedly *never* used deodorants or antiperspirants in their lifetime. What this tells us is that parabens, regardless of the source, can bioaccumulate in breast tissue. And the sources are many. Parabens can be found in a wide variety of personal care products, cosmetics, as well as drugs. That said, it appears the *dermal route* is the most significant form of exposure. Another component of antiperspirants, aluminum chloride, has been found to act similarly to the way oncogenes work to provide molecular transformations in cancer cells.

Other Breast Cancer Prevention Strategies

In the largest review of research into lifestyle and breast cancer, the American Institute of Cancer Research estimated that about 40 percent of US breast cancer cases could be prevented if people made wiser lifestyle choices. I believe these are low-ball estimates. More than likely, 75 percent to 90 percent of breast cancers could be avoided by strictly applying lifestyle modifications.

11 Surprising Reasons Organic Is Better for You

Ever find yourself eyeing up the organic label, wondering if it's actually worth it. According to a huge new review study published in the *British Journal of Nutrition*, it is. With the latest study offering even more proof that organic is the best choice, we wanted to share some of the more intriguing reasons buying organic protects your body (and the planet)!

#1: More antioxidants. Organic fruits and vegetables contain 20 to 40 percent more disease-fighting antioxidants compared to chemically grown counterparts. In fact, eating only organic food is equivalent to eating an extra serving of fruit or veggies a day, without actually having to eat more food.

#2: Lower poisonous metal levels. Organic food is up to 48 percent lower the metal cadmium, a toxic compound found in certain fertilizers. It's also linked to breast cancer and kidney stones.

#3: More healthy plant compounds. Plants exposed to pesticides produce fewer natural pest defenses, including phenols and polyphenols, naturally occurring compounds that can protect your organs and lower anxiety levels. Organic plants boast much higher flavonoid levels, in some cases up to around 70 percent higher levels.

#4: Fewer chemicals inside of food. It's not enough to wash your nonorganic veggies. Many chemicals are systemic, meaning they're taken up inside of the plants that we eat. In fact, a recent Norwegian study found we're actually eating levels of Roundup.

#5: Better fat. A 2013 study found that organic milk is higher in brain- and heart-healthy omega-3 fatty acids, thanks in part to spending more time out on pasture, a requirement in organics. Not only did nonorganic milk contain lower levels of the good fats, but it also harbored higher levels of dangerous inflammatory fats.

#6: Fewer superbugs. About 90,000 lives are lost each year to antibiotic-resistant superbug infections. Where are these dangerous germs coming from? Many nonorganic farms feed low-dose antibiotics to their animals daily to speed growth and get the animal to slaughter sooner. The trouble is, germs exposed to drugs regularly are able to outsmart the drugs. (And often, they're even hiding out on the meat you bring home from the supermarket!) You're more than 30 percent less likely to come in contact with superbugs in the meat supply when you choose organic.

#7: Food NOT grown in human sewage sludge. It's perfectly legal for nonorganic farmers to douse nonorganic fields with human sewage sludge taken from municipal water treatment plants as fertilizer for their crops. The sludge could contain whatever morgues, residences, and industrial parks decide to put down the drain. Scientists have detected shampoo chemicals in nonorganic tomatoes and hypothesize that sewage sludge is partly to blame.

#8: Protection from weird food additives. Organic has a clear health advantage when it comes to packaged foods, too. Instead of harmful artificial food dyes linked to brain cell damage and ADHD, organic food processors turn to natural colorings like beet juice to give products a desired color.

#9: Cleaner rain. Nonorganic farmers use so much glyphosate, the main ingredient in Roundup, that government scientists have now detected it in the rain! Even tiny amounts of America's most popular weed killer can damage DNA and kill cells, and they've been linked to infertility and certain cancers.

#10: Better for the bees. If you want access to healthy food, you need pollinators. But mounting research is pointing to neonicotinoid insecticides as a leading cause of colony collapse disorder. These toxic, brain-damaging insecticides are banished in organics.

#11. A healthier climate. According to studies done on soil science, if all the cropland on Earth were treated organically, the soil would sequester 41 percent of all the greenhouse gases in the atmosphere; pastureland could sequester an **additional** 71 percent! If just half the world's cropland and pastureland were converted, organic soil could pull 55 percent of annual carbon emissions out of the atmosphere.

Feel free to email Doug at DCaporrino@yahoo.com or
visit his website http://www.Dougcaporrino.com

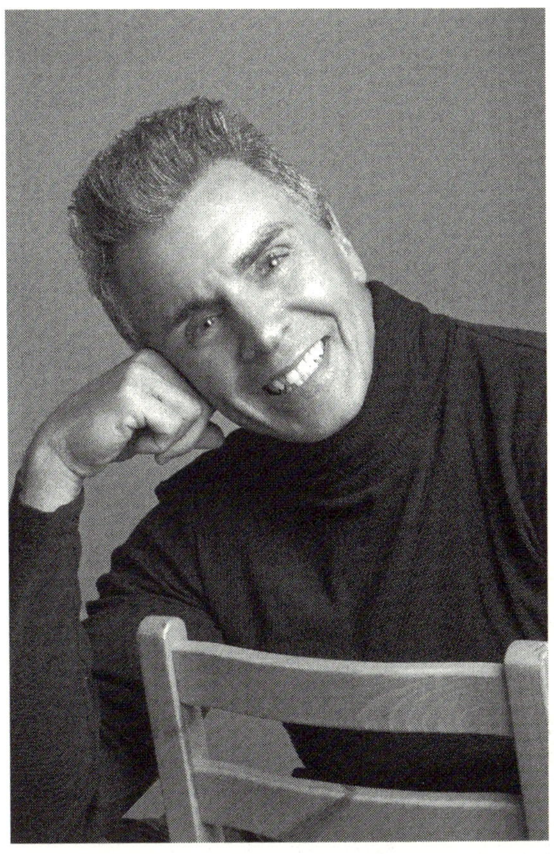

Douglas Caporrino has been peeling back the layers of the onion for the better part of his life. Taking control of his own health challenges from an early age, he has never accepted one, two or even three opinions. He researches daily and looks at all the whys, what, when and hows, so you don't have to. He has helped countless people through his years of lecturing all over the world, wellness coaching, diagnostic testing, and common-sense approach to growing young. No one should have to suffer in life with their health given the knowledge and know how that is available today.

Every single disease can be traced back to a nutritional deficiency in your body. Let Doug help you find that deficiency.